32.50

D1426760

Doing good?

Psychotherapy out of its depth

Doing good?

Psychotherapy out of its depth

Peter Lomas

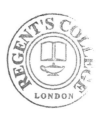

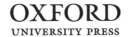

OXFORD
UNIVERSITY PRESS

OXFORD
UNIVERSITY PRESS

Great Clarendon Street, Oxford OX2 6DP

Oxford University Press is a department of the University of Oxford
and furthers the University's aim of excellence in research, scholarship,
and education by publishing worldwide in

Oxford New York

Athens Auckland Bangkok Bogotá Buenos Aires Calcutta
Cape Town Chennai Dar es Salaam Delhi Florence Hong Kong Istanbul
Karachi Kuala Lumpur Madrid Melbourne Mexico City Mumbai
Nairobi Paris São Paulo Singapore Taipei Tokyo Toronto Warsaw

with associated companies in Berlin Ibadan

Oxford is a trade mark of Oxford University Press
in the UK and in certain other countries

Published in the United States
by Oxford University Press Inc., New York

British Library Cataloguing in Publication Data

Data available

Library of Congress Cataloging in Publication Data
Lomas, Peter.
Doing good?: Psychotherapy out of its depth / Peter Lomas.
P.   cm.
Includes index
1. Psychotherapist and patient. 2. Psychotherapy—Philosophy.
3. Psychotherapy—Moral and ethical aspects. I. Title.
RC480.5.L587   1999 616.89'14'01—dc21   99–34797

ISBN 0 19 262868 2

1 3 5 7 9 10 8 6 4 2

Typeset in Meridien
by Alliance Phototypesetters, Pondicherry, India
Printed in Great Britain
on acid-free paper by
Biddles Ltd., Guildford & King's Lynn

With my Gauloise dying out,
Over a glass of red wine,
I muse on the meaning of being this and not that.

From *What Does It Mean* Czeslaw Milosz

Contents

Contents

1

How should we live?

If you tell me that you would at this moment have a fig, I will answer you that there must be time. Let it first blossom, then bear fruit, then ripen. Is then the fruit of a fig-tree not brought to perfection suddenly, in one hour; and would you possess the fruit of the human mind in so short a time, and without trouble? I tell you, expect no such thing.

Epictetus

There has never been a shortage of people ready to tell others how to live. Sometimes such advice comes from someone who is regarded as having particular knowledge in a certain field of operations, and, if luck holds, the advice will be helpful. But what of advice that is of a more general nature? In most of daily living this comes from relatives, friends, and the man-in-the-street, that is, those who cannot be expected to know the answers any better than we ourselves, whose opinions may be unsought and unwelcome, yet to whom we might gratefully turn when in distress. By contrast, there are the prophets and sages, those who, for one reason or another, have acquired a reputation for wisdom. Most of them are dead; and it is a brave, stupid, or foolhardy person who will readily stand up in the market-place and claim to be wise. Yet, in effect, this is what the psychotherapist is called upon to do.

It is rare for someone to approach the therapist with the questions: 'How should I live?' or 'What shall I do to be saved?'

But the experience of distress will almost certainly involve questions of how to act or think about certain matters, and the more these matters are explored the more they will be seen to shift over into the broader issues of living. And, if a sage were to hand, he or she would seem to be the best person to help out.

If there is any truth in the scenario that I depict then the psychotherapist is in an extremely uncomfortable position. He is torn between an attempt to fulfil the role into which he has been placed—that is to say, to speak with wisdom—or to ensure on the other hand that his words are uncontaminated by anything that could possibly be considered to be advice from a superior being. The usual consequence is that he falls between two stools; he fudges the issue. This, to my mind, is one of the reasons—possibly the main reason—why contemporary psychotherapy is in a state of flux. One way of attempting to bypass this dilemma is for the psychotherapist to claim to possess a technique which is not the product of - wisdom, yet, for some reason or another, appears to help troubled people. A rationale is usually given for its efficacy, which, in our age, is articulated in terms of scientific method. Later in the book (Chapter 5), I shall offer some reasons why I think that the contemporary trust in technique is misplaced.

Today, although the methods most favoured by the health service in Britain are those derived from experimental psychology, there is no doubt that, for the last century, the most influential ideas on the subject have been those of Sigmund Freud; and despite the waning reputation of orthodox psychoanalysis, this remains the case. Freud laid no claim to wisdom. He saw his task as that of bringing to light the hidden reasons for the patient's distress, using a method that he had devised himself. To the extent that he was successful in this aim he restored to the patient the capacity to take a greater responsibility for his own life and make more informed decisions. Among his followers, Schafer[1] is prominent in spelling out the ways in which a 'neurotic' person avoids taking responsibility: the psychoanalyst's aim is to unravel the confusions that prevent purposeful and realistic action.

This formula has an ancient and formidable pedigree. As Roger Scruton notes:

The philosopher, in Plato's characterisation, awakens the spirit of enquiry. He helps his listeners to discover the truth, and it is they who bring forth, under his catalysing influence, the answer to life's riddles. The philosopher is the midwife, and his duty is to help us be what we are—free and rational beings, who lack nothing that is required to understand our condition.[2]

Following this path, Freud greatly increased our appreciation of the difficulties of achieving self-knowledge and suggested ways in which a block to insight could be resolved. Countless numbers of people can now pay tribute to the efficacy of his project, and the search for such understanding remains paramount for those who he has influenced. One of the limitations of his endeavour, however, is that in systemizing his observations, he limited a free and open exploration of 'the answer to life's riddles'. The confusions to be unravelled are seen in the light of his system of thought. The 'true' picture of the world, which the patient has lost, is assumed to be that expressed by the therapist's formula. There is no reason to explore it. There is no need to discuss the question of what would constitute a valuable life for the patient.

Although, as I have suggested, it is rare for someone to start his therapy with the question: 'How should I live?' he may well say something which implies: 'Can you help me to manage my life better?' or 'I don't know how to be?' or 'I don't feel I know how to get through the day?' The person who conveys his plight in such words is concerned with value. 'Is life worth living? What is worth doing? Other people seem to get a kick out of life; why can't I?' These questions have a moral resonance.

In contemporary moral philosophy—and indeed in daily speech—the term 'moral' is usually given a rather narrow focus—the compliance or not to a code of conduct that can be defined with some degree of certainty: an action is either right or wrong. But morality has not always been so defined. In *The morality of happiness*,[3] Julia Annas charts a significant change between ancient and modern ethical concepts. The Greeks did not base their thinking on the idea that morality is punitive or corrective: they did not assume, as do the majority of contemporary thinkers, that a moral life is one that is harassed and persecuted everywhere by imperatives and disagreeable duties. 'Its leading notions', Annas maintains, are not those of obligation, duty and rule-following; instead of these "imperative" notions it uses attractive notions like those of goodness and worth. Ancient ethical theories do not assume that morality is essentially demanding, the only interesting question being, how much does it demand, rather the moral point of view is seen as one that the agent will naturally come to accept in the course of a normal unrepressed development.[4]

It is in the sense conceived by Annas that I shall use the term 'morality' in what follows, and the issue that I want to raise centres on the idea that our contemporary model of psycho-therapeutic endeavour is quite remarkable in that it omits the moral dimension of living. Once we allow that aspect of ex-perience into our thinking, many awkward questions emerge. On what authority does the therapist make a claim for know-ing what constitutes a good life? What place, if any, does tech-nique have in an encounter which takes place in a moral world? May the moral attributes shown by the therapist in the room be more significant than anything else? What does it mean to behave well in therapy? Is the therapist's aim to help the patient towards health (whatever that is) or is it to enable him to be a better person? Finally (though not exhaustively): is there a moral choice in becoming ill? Even if we take the ex-treme case of schizophrenia—a mental illness *par excellence*—there can be doubt about the matter. Sass describes a schizophrenic patient whom he treated, who said that,

he knew he would not have become ill if he had not made the mis-take, at the outset of the psychotic break, of sitting back and watch-ing his friends at a party instead of joining in their activities; only then, he explained, have things looked "weird". This kind of correla-tion between particular modes of activity (or inactivity) and certain forms of experience suggests that the experiences in question could perhaps be controlled, at least in part, through the adoption of one or another stance or mode of activity.[5]

It is now a widely accepted fact—argued by innumerable thinkers over the past century or so—that, in the West at least, religion has been largely displaced by a reliance on science and technique. Technique, moreover, has expanded from a method of controlling things to the control of ways of living. That this change has proved hazardous if not disastrous to the physical world is not in doubt and the consequences to the world of human relations may well have suffered comparable disruption and corruption. In view of this hazard, can any area of living, including psychotherapy, continue to accept the centrality of technique without question?

Language, however rich, is a frail vehicle for conveying our experience of living and there are few areas of our life in which this inadequacy manifests itself so sharply as that of morality; a fact which helps to explain why psychotherapists tend to avoid the use of this word—or, indeed, any word with similar connotations—when talking about their theory and practice, and find themselves more at ease in thinking of their work as a method which is defined in a circumscribed way. However, as Freeman Dyson writes:

There is no such thing as a unique scientific vision, any more than there is a unique poetic vision. Science is a mosaic of partial and conflicting visions. But there is one common element in these visions. The common element is rebellion against the restrictions imposed by the locally prevailing culture, Western or Eastern as the case may be.[6]

Dyson's view of science is an attractive one. It is broad. The science against which the contemporary psychotherapist has to struggle in finding an acceptable voice is limited to a Procrustean bed of technical procedures and quantitative measurements. The therapist who wishes to be heard with respect may easily feel that he or she must keep quiet about any ideas which do not fit this 'locally prevailing culture'. One such idea is that the therapist's aims are concerned with the moral betterment of the lives of those who come for help. If we take Dyson's view seriously, the true 'scientific vision' should be able to incorporate this fact. But we are a long way from such a view. Science and morality are uneasy bedfellows: morality is a very personal matter and the current scientific vision does not take kindly to the personal.

In this century, the personal has come under attack from quite a different quarter. The terms 'modernism' and 'postmodernism', although centred on art forms, are also used to incorporate our whole culture. The personal view of the world, that which gives meaning and coherence to experience, has been savagely undermined, fragmented, or articulated with ironic overtones in recent years. It is a paradox that in an age when so much attention is given to the personal (to the extent that we are dubbed the 'me generation') the value of personal experience and personal ideas of morality are so threatened and suspect. To what degree, and in what way, does the prevailing devaluation of the personal inform the contemporary concepts and practice of psychotherapy? This is a question I shall address in the next chapter.

One of the many difficulties which besets psychotherapy is that one has either to accept the basic premises of living of one school of thought (that derived from Freud being by far the most influential) or one has to look elsewhere, in unfamiliar areas. Few of us are trained in psychology, sociology, anthropology, literature, child development, theology, philosophy, or other relevant disciplines, nor can we claim any expertise in ordinary living. Yet, if we are to escape from too narrow a focus we have to take account of these areas; and one area which cries out to be explored is that of ethics. I am not simply referring to the problems which arise when therapists breach certain codes of conduct laid down by a professional authority but the way in which the attempt to heal a human being is pervaded by, even defined by, our value system. To introduce moral values is not to suggest a few adjustments here and there to our methods, but to question the method itself. This does not mean, however, that we have to discard the invaluable insights which psychotherapy has already brought. To put the matter a different way, it is less a question of incorporating moral issues into the framework of analytical psychotherapy than of shifting the paradigm of our work in such a way that these issues no longer take a back seat.

A major consequence of the Freudian revolution is that those who minister to our psychic frailties find it less easy to bring us to our senses by means of fear. They can no longer speak with massive authority of the known and certain paths of righteousness, to stray from which will bring everlasting misery. Sex is no longer sinful, and wickedness itself is no longer a frightening evil force that enters from without, but is part and parcel of our natural selves. This assertion is, of course, a gross oversimplification. Freud did not, to say the least, manage the change all on his own; the forces that have brought about our present state are infinitely complex. And the psychiatrist can, in his own way and with his own language, still frighten us to death. But the achievement stands— and we do not want to lose it. This, I believe, is one reason why psychotherapy presents itself as free from the moral dimension. The patient comes and the therapist listens with rigorous care and thought, looking especially for clues to experiences that are beyond the patient's conscious knowledge. He does not comment on the patient's moral condition or sermonize on what is right or wrong behaviour: he merely encourages him to find his own voice, and in order to help him do this he pieces together, as best he can, the arguments, contradictions, distortions, evasions, and silences, and then constructs an account which is both coherent and commensurate with reality. The very fact that he does not make moral judgements, that he accepts the patient's admissions of feebleness, sinfulness, and despair with serenity and compassion, enables the latter to reveal his failures more easily and to respect himself in spite of them.

How can we criticize, let alone abandon, a method that has so much to commend it? We may disagree with some of the pronouncements of Freud and those who have followed him. We may deplore the exaggerations, the rigidities, and the stupidities of certain practitioners and groups. Yet the main thrust of this approach is so humane and contains so much wisdom and has unveiled so much useful knowledge about the human psyche that it claims our support. Let us not look this gift-horse in the mouth, we might be tempted to say, and let us focus on our strong suit, interpretation. It is a seductive line of thought but it may confine us too much to the safe and known paths. If psychotherapy were simply a matter of helping the patient to trace thoughts, feelings, and memories of which he is unaware, then the therapist's ethical views have no bearing on the undertaking. Critiques of the technique of the psychotherapist are usually made on the basis of whether it is a good or bad technique. The question as to whether it is ethical to use a technique is not addressed. Yet to practise a technique on a patient is to say to him, in effect: 'This is how I am going to behave towards you. I will hope to do so with sensitivity and compassion, and I will certainly have your good in mind. But I shall stick to this technique, whether you like it or not, because this is how I believe psychotherapy should be done. The matter is not negotiable.'

There are two problems with this stance. First, is it ethical for one person to dictate the form in which a relationship will take place? There would have to be a very good reason for such an unequal partnership and it is doubtful whether psychotherapy can produce one. Secondly, although what in practice takes place in such an arrangement may well, most of the time, appear ethically inoffensive, one can easily imagine cases in which a therapist may, while following what he believes to be a correct technique, act unethically. For example, should one, in the interests of neutrality, do nothing to stop a patient killing himself? And if a therapist charges the patient a fee when the latter misses a session because of illness (which is a common practice) does he do so in order that the patient will be unable to feign illness as a form of resistance to therapy or does he do so because he wants the money? It may be perfectly legitimate to demand the money but not to be hypocritical about the reason for so doing.

If the technique under consideration is one that is derived from psychoanalytic thinking interpretation will be its main *raison d'être*. But we now face a further problem, for interpretations are not made in an ethical vacuum. The therapist's views on almost every issue involving personal relations will influence whether he interprets a particular statement, whether he remains silent, or whether he expresses agreement. It is simply not possible for him to shed his sense of values when he enters the consulting room however much he may try to do so. Written accounts of work reveal this fact: the most telling way in which the therapist reveals his sense of how he believes people should behave is his actual behaviour to the patient.

The fact that, as noted above, the declared aim of psychoanalysis is to restore or engender a sense of personal responsibility is itself an affirmation of a certain virtue. Freud himself was a man of definite views on morality as has been shown by many writers, including Riesman,[7] Rieff,[8] and Roazen,[9] and his views had a direct bearing on the interpretations he made to his patients. It is manifestly absurd for Freud, or for any psychotherapist to lay claim to moral neutrality. The possibilities of proselytizing are frightening. I sometimes have the fantasy that the most appropriate sign a psychotherapist could hang on his door would be 'Do Not Trust Me'.

If it is the case that the therapist cannot fail to reveal his ethical predilections and thereby influence patients in their direction it would, I believe, be better to confront this matter quite openly as a problem that cannot be evaded. And if he is bound to influence patients it is best that the influence be a good one. How can this be accomplished? It is a daunting task, for therapists are not moral giants. The most reasonable way of tackling this dilemma is not only to ensure that therapists discuss ethical matters much more than they do at present but that they be prepared to discuss them with their patients on the basis of equality—that is to say, claiming no priority of knowledge in this area and being prepared to admit their doubt and possible bias. Psychoanalysis has an unhealthy history of either ignoring ideas that do not fit the theory, or trying to absorb them into its orbit without a radical theoretical change; and this, in part, may account for the silence on the matter. When ethical issues erupt, as for example, the sexual seduction of patients by therapists, the profession is prepared to recognize that there is a problem, but it is regarded as an aberration which does not concern normal day-to-day practice.

Once we give much more attention to the question of the psychotherapist's moral stance than we do at present, many questions inevitably follow. What results does the therapist aim for? A better person? A happier person? A more adaptive person? And in what moral terms does he see his own participation—a profession or a calling? Questions of these kinds lead on to the perennial dilemma: what is therapeutic in the exercise? What really helps people? If intellectual understanding is not enough, then what heals? Is it care? Despite the recognition of the therapeutic value of love by Ferenczi,[10] Suttie,[11] and many others, the question of the goodness and decency of the therapist is still not confronted intellectually by the profession. Goodness is taken for granted and quickly forgotten (despite the fact that psychoanalysts explore both their individual negative feelings and the narcissistic motives behind the choice of profession), for it is an embarrassment to those who wish to escape the dismissive label of 'do-gooders'. Yet, if the flow of life is extinguished when the patient lacks a sense of value, it is difficult to see how the therapist can do otherwise than give care, in the ways that seem most appropriate in the circumstances, and give it not because of a theory or professional pride, but from a genuine emotion. This does not mean that it is a thoughtless care, that the therapist will necessarily do what the patient asks, but that, given his experience and knowledge and whatever qualities he possesses, he will endeavour to offer whatever help he can, accepting the limits of what is reasonable to provide. I realize that in saying this I am in danger of presenting the therapist as a saint and the consulting room as a haven of peace and amicability. But I have no such illusions. If what happens is good the reason is to be found, I believe, not in any exceptional virtue in the therapist but in an unusual situation that, fortuitously, can engender a virtuous relationship.

The stuff of life cannot be well conveyed discursively. If philosophy could do it we would have no need of art. The reporting of an event is primarily done by people who are neither philosophers nor artists, but who were there and can testify from their perceptions. If, however, the reporter can bring a degree of art and intellectual understanding of the event the reader will be the richer. Many psychotherapists have a wish to convey the nature and experience of their work to others. This is done both by theoretical formulations and what are usually called 'case-histories'. But how well do the latter communicate what really goes on in the room? Less, I believe, than we like to think. Case-histories consist of stories written about one person by another who formulates them according to a general theory of illness and its cure; the patient's contribution is limited to those of his utterances considered to be relevant to the theory. Although much has been learnt by such means, it is a very restricted vision. A psychotherapist may be unsure of his capacity to write a good case-history but does not readily question whether the undertaking itself is suspect. For those who doubt this, who believe, as I do, that therapy is best conceived and achieved in terms of a conversation between two people, a further problem appears. How can one justify the reporting of a conversation as though it were purporting to communicate an insight into the nature of therapy unless it is done under the aegis of a general theory? What is the use of simply reporting the conversation and leaving it at that? Surely, we might just as well report a conversation on a bus and claim it is of more significance than any other of the myriad conversations that constitute social life? We can, however, say that we are reporting a particular kind of conversation that occurs when someone attempts to help another in circumstances that are different from those which occur in the course of everyday living. This, I think, is its main justification.

The better the listener or the better the writer, the greater chance the reader is given to use his own wit to understand what is going on. Each therapist will bring his or her own beliefs, experiences and preconceptions to the room, and these will colour the conversations, but this is an inevitable restriction to all reporting. An account that is as unselected a presentation of what was said and felt as can be managed is, however, likely to bring some illumination. The task is not unlike that of the novelist who records imaginary conversations. But his or her justification for their work rests on literary skill for which the psychotherapist has no claim. 'On seeking guidance on how to live,' writes Martha Nussbaum,[12] 'we turn to stories of practical wisdom, both for representations of fine attention and in order to be formed ourselves, as readers, into just such attentive and discriminating beings.' In other words, the novelist (and Nussbaum has in mind the novelist of genius) can pay attention to any portion of life and record it, through an imaginative mode of discourse, with such insight and perspicacity that the reader is enlightened as to what is and what can be. Ideally, such a gift could be fruitfully used to describe the factual experience of a psychotherapeutic encounter. Although therapists lack that gift, they can aspire to such an aim and, if they are any good at their work, they have probably learnt to be attentive to nuances.

There are many factors which stand in the way of a satisfying description of therapeutic experience. The anonymity of the patient must be preserved; some conversations are simply too private to be disclosed, even if disguised; and if therapy goes badly wrong it is not easy to obtain the patient's permission to describe it; and however good the account, what we get for the most part, are the words spoken and not the tone of voice or the expression in the eyes. It is all too clear that the reader is getting a poor bargain. A further problem is the sheer banality that occurs in actual conversations of any kind and which is bound to occur in any description of therapy that does not centre on technique. If, for example, in a session the patient breaks off to say: 'That pneumatic drill is making a hell of a noise' and the therapist replies: 'Yes, it is. They're doing it all week. Something to do with the drains', should this natural but rather trivial interchange be recorded or not. Yet, if we omit it, the flavour of the relationship is altered. In what follows, I have chosen, when describing conversations in therapy, to set down what was actually said insofar as I can remember. These short vignettes are selected, consciously, to illustrate certain themes. No doubt they will have been selected unconsciously for all kinds of reasons, not least the desire to sound respectable. The subtlety with which we can portray ourselves in a decent garb even when aiming to be unadorned can hardly be overestimated (the Devil is a master at enabling us to preserve our narcissism). I hope, however, that by deliberately including the prosaic and apparently inconsequential, I give the reader a better chance of coming to his or her own conclusions. In the same way that novelists and poets try to articulate how one might best live because there is no formula that can encapsulate life, psychotherapists need, I believe, to find a richer vehicle than jargon because there is no formula to summarize their work.

I seem to have managed to concoct an impressive list of excuses for the inadequacy of the brief conversations I describe in this book. But my apologies are still not complete; I have yet another. If what is recorded by a psychotherapist is not the application of a technique, then it is an account of what he or she is personally like in the consulting room. His or her style of being is on display, even if transmitted only by a series of glimpses. I can hardly parade my own as something admirable. Its inclusion therefore is not to be taken as an example of good therapy except, perhaps, for the occasions when I am hoping to suggest that departing from accepted technique is not necessarily disastrous and may even be helpful. There would probably be general agreement that intelligence and sensitivity are important qualities in a practitioner. We can take this for granted and need not talk about it. But there are other qualities which I seek to justify in this book that are more open to debate and therefore need to be debated. One of these, which I discuss in the next chapter, is ordinariness. Insofar as this quality has some similarity to what we call 'the common touch' or 'naturalness', I am in trouble. To claim to possess it is as outrageous and futile as to claim a sense of humour. And, indeed, the question of humour is also central to any conception of ordinariness. Joking rarely makes an appearance in the case-histories and conversations recounted by psychotherapists and this gives them a solemnity and aridity which, I suspect, does not accurately reflect the tone of many real encounters. My own analyst, Charles Rycroft, had a wonderfully dry sense of humour which he often shared with me and I sometimes think this did me as much good as his rigorous interpretations. But humorous comments of that kind do not appear in his published case-histories, and, I regret, I have not had the nerve to quote more than one or two of my own in what follows. Psychotherapists, I guess, are not only, like others, afraid of exhibiting their capacity for humour in the form of examples but are keen to avoid the appearance of being superficial or flippant in the face of distress—an absurd thought, for the distressed need it more than most.

Those of us who have learnt much from Freud find it difficult, if not impossible, to escape his grasp. We wear his clothes—not because we want to but because they are the clothes in our wardrobes. There is a danger of writing negatively, of spelling out the ways in which Freud was wrong or limited rather than moving forward on new paths, of rejecting insights so useful that we are impoverished by their loss. This is the kind of dilemma that confronts all disciplines whose history contains thinkers of the first order, but one is seldom faced with a practice that is so permeated by the ideas of its originator as is psychotherapy. While valuing certain of Freud's ideas we need to be circumspect about those that are contrary to ordinary good sense at its best and traditions of thought which have, with justification, been handed down to us over the centuries, many if not all of which can only be properly articulated in ordinary language and which implicitly include moral visions of living.

Although, in this book, I am making a plea for the moral element of living to be fully recognized by psychotherapy I am not proposing that psychotherapy is encapsulated by the word 'moral'. Indeed, I find it difficult to think of any word, or arrangement of words, adequate to conceive the nature of the work. The meaning of the term 'psychotherapy' is so elusive and so unsatisfactory that its very use misleads people into thinking there is something around, called by this name, that has a solid foundation and can be accurately formulated, as, for example, the word 'elephant'. I sometimes wish we could get rid of the word altogether. But it is here to stay for a while in order to identify the practice of those who counsel people in distress and publicly profess it to be their work.

References

1. Schafer, R. (1976). *A new language for psychoanalysis*. Yale University Press, New Haven, CT.
2. Scruton, R. (1997). The return of the sophist. *The Times*, 11 August.
3. Annas, J. (1993). *The morality of happiness*. Oxford University Press.
4. Annas, J. (1993). Op. cit.
5. Sass, L. (1992). *Madness and modernism. Insanity in the light of modern art, literature and thought*, pp. 72–3. Harvard University Press, Cambridge, MA.
6. Dyson, F. (1995). The scientist as rebel. *New York Review of Books*, 25 May, 31.
7. Riesman, D. (1954). *Individualism reconsidered*. The Free Press, New York.
8. Rieff, P. (1965). *Freud: The mind of the moralist*. Methuen, London.
9. Roazen, P. (1968). *Freud: Political and social thought*. Knopf, New York.
10. Ferenczi, S. (1988). *The clinical diary of Sandor Ferenczi*, (ed. S. Dupont, trans. M. Balint and N. Z. Jackson). Harvard University Press, Cambridge, MA.
11. Suttie, I. (1988). *The origins of love and hate*. Free Association Books, London.
12. Nussbaum, M. (1990). *Love's knowledge: Essays on philosophy and literature*. Oxford University Press.

2

The retreat from the ordinary

Those who are unhappy have no need for anything in this world but people capable of giving them their attention. The capacity to give one's attention to a sufferer is a very rare and difficult thing. It is almost a miracle; it is a miracle.

Simone Weil

If a person is troubled in her heart and cannot see any avenue of escape from her emotional turmoil it would make good sense to seek help from someone who has a reputation for being of use in such matters. The prospective helper may be a wise person or an expert. By expert, I mean someone who has at their disposal a particular ploy, tactic, technique, procedure, or trick upon which they would rely to ease the supplicant's torment; such a ploy may or may not involve an illusion. In some cultures a technique used for such a purpose would be thought of as magic or religious and involve supernatural powers; today, we would be more likely to look for an explanation in the natural world, one which we would attribute to what we call 'science'. There has, however, always been a confusion between wisdom and technique. As anthropologists have noted, the shaman who enacts a magical ritual or who pretends (and perhaps even believes) that it is efficacious may use whatever common sense or wisdom he or she possesses in order to solve the problem.

The contemporary psychotherapist purports to rely, for the most part, on technique. In saying this, I do not mean to imply that the technique is necessarily a deception or may not be efficacious. Its purpose is to persuade, enlighten, convince, teach, stimulate, encourage, or jolt someone into a change for the better, and the ploys may or may not depend on the power of suggestion. Asan,[1] in a paper in which he deplores the excessive prevalence of techniques in family therapy, gives an example of 'solution-focused' work, a technique which, although 'simplified to a degree that is almost embarrassing', nevertheless can sometimes be useful. This model is based on the observation that symptoms and problems have a tendency to fluctuate. The family is encouraged to focus on situations in which the member exhibiting the symptom—say, depression—is in a good phase, and to amplify all the factors which were present during these good situations.

The psychoanalyst or analytical therapist also uses ploys ('Lie on the couch, say what comes into your head, but don't expect an answer to your questions', etc.); but, from Freud onwards, there has been a recognition in the analytic school of thought that therapy consists not of an odd jolt here and an argument there, but a confrontation of the whole being of the person, an understanding of his life in depth. This attitude involves asking the question: 'How can I help this person to lead a better life? What is a good life?' We are now in different territory from that of technique for we now need a wise person, someone who knows about the depths of experience, or, at least, someone who is prepared to enter a conversation about wisdom. The psychotherapist who works with this approach is in danger of confusion. She proclaims that she relies on a technique, yet knows that what is also required, and perhaps even what is most required—the *sine qua non* of her endeavour—is her capacity, from everything she has learnt in life, to understand in her heart, the experience of the other person and to respond with wisdom, compassion, intelligence, and honesty. Can these two approaches be combined in the same practitioner? Do we have to make a choice between either: (a) 'I offer a method for change. Don't expect me to know about life or have any wisdom', or (b) 'I have no method and no theory. I have decided to offer myself as someone to talk to about life problems; and I have gained some experience of doing this and I seem to have been of some use to some people'?

The problem with the former approach is that it appears to be insufficient to come near to the depths of individual human experience and pain. The problem with the latter is the difficulty of justifying a claim to being wise enough for the job—a claim which seems to imply an absurd and arrogant belief in the possession of superior wisdom. But is it really the case that such a claim is inevitably an arrogant one? Someone may simply, for whatever reason, have a desire to do this particular kind of work and find that he or she is sufficiently good at it, after receiving whatever help is available to them, to justify inviting others into their consulting room—that is to say, into a setting which facilitates whatever wisdom he or she happens to possess. But such a person would not be a psychotherapist in the sense in which the word is understood in our society. To claim to be a psychotherapist today implies adherence to a particular school of thought and method. As David Smail comments:

It is really quite difficult for most people even to imagine a concept of "truth" which is not tied so closely into some kind of discipline as to be more or less identical with it.[2]

There is a further phenomenon to take into consideration. Those who now seek help for psychic disturbance usually present their problem in a very different way from those who consulted Freud. They are less likely to show hysterical paralysis or comparable isolated symptoms with a medical feel to them. They do not say, for example, 'I get a pain in my head and pass out whenever I see a politician on television'. What is more likely is that they will say something to the effect that they are lost, unhappy, confused, inhibited, anxious, unworthy, or have a problem in their relations with others. Leaving aside the reasons for this change (which may include the work of Freud himself) their plight comes in terms which might in the past have been considered the province of the priest. And we may be justified, therefore, in thinking that an appropriate response today may well be different from the one advocated by Freud. To put it another way, although Freud attempted to rescue the distressed from religion and offer a better alternative, we now may have to offer a better alternative

than science as understood by Freud. It is likely that many
therapists today do in fact rely on compassion and wisdom, but
we are a very long way from being able to articulate this convincingly. If we address this matter at all, we fall back on gen-
eralizations such as 'love heals' or 'psychotherapy is an art';
and, however true such statements may be, they do not take
us very far.

Despite the distortions inherent in psychoanalysis, we have
learnt a lot about helping people from this discipline in the last
hundred years. Practitioners of the art of alleviating emotional
distress have been having conversations with those in anguish
to an unprecedented degree. Much has been thought about
and recorded. Many of the men and women undertaking this
task have been good, rigorous, responsible, and wise and have
much to teach us despite the fact that their message is often
obscured by an esoteric language that would make George
Orwell turn in his grave. Even if we were to say, for the sake of
argument, that their technique and theory wasn't worth a
penny, much of value has been gained and it would be very
foolish to dismiss their experience.

What we have yet to do is to find some way of describing
psychotherapy that coherently incorporates the practical wisdom involved in it without losing the special experience
gained from the genius of Freud, what has developed from
Freud, and what is valuable in other systemized approaches.
In other words, it is quite legitimate to use Freud's insights
even while we reject the methods by which he gained them
and the superstructure of theory in which they are embedded.
Moreover, the degree to which Freud's insights derived from
his method (as he claimed) is now uncertain.

What constitutes everyday, ordinary ways of thinking is dependent on the culture of a particular time and place. In previous centuries the assumptions of Christianity were taken for
granted. People went to church and there were experts in theology, but the man-in-the-street did not have to go to a practitioner to learn ideas that were already part of his social
environment. Today, we take the assumptions of science for
granted; we do not need special tuition in the theory that the
earth is round. And educated people have heard of Freud and
are familiar with the view, say, that repressed anger can often
be seen to account for certain behaviour. Although Freud had

some rather novel ideas to teach those who came to him for help, psychotherapists often do not have to labour the point or introduce a complicated technique to demonstrate the phenomena.

Although it would seem to make sense to think of psychotherapy as a situation which heals by facilitating care and wisdom yet can be greatly enriched by what has been learnt in the psychoanalytic tradition, I suspect that in the present climate of opinion any hint of an amalgamation of two very different paradigms would fail to take us beyond the present muddle, in which lip service is given to the value of ordinary qualities in the therapist while the essence of the work is located in theory and technique. One reason for this is that it is very much easier to formulate a technique than it is to articulate the nature of wise behaviour; attempts to do the latter can very easily sound naïve or vague.

A radical revision of what we consider to be the basis of our work would involve changes in thought and practice that one can hardly bear to confront. It would require a complete rethinking of training and the organization of psychotherapy, for, if theory and technique were no longer considered the essence of the work, we could not require students to learn it and would have to find another way of easing the path of those who wish to offer their help to people in mental distress. I believe that today such a move would be unacceptable. Psychotherapy is in a condition rather like that of a patient whose defensive character is so rigid that the therapist has the limited aim of helping the person to live a life that is slightly less crippled by defences. It may be that, for the present, this is all we can hope for, or, at the very least, that we may halt the plunge into an even greater reliance on technical expertise— an outcome which, at present, seems the likely consequence of the registration of psychotherapy.

Psychotherapists are, of course, not alone in this kind of predicament. It is endemic to our age. We have retreated into specialization. It is easier to say what we have retreated into than what we have retreated from, for the negative is usually simpler to formulate than the positive. Possible ways of putting it are to say that the retreat is from 'ordinary' living or from 'full' living, but I am aware that such phrases convey little. In using them I am asserting a belief or faith that there are ways of living that are better than others, and that the reader's idea of what is good, in the broadest sense, has sufficient similarity to my own for us to usefully talk to each other. I am thinking of fundamental issues rather than details. For example, I believe it is good to perceive the world in a way that corresponds sufficiently with its actuality to get us through the day without being taken to a mental hospital, that it is better that one is not crippled by unrealistic fear, consumed by murderous hate, or is a persistent liar or seducer.

There are many ways of describing a retreat from full living. Every age has its own particular mode of retreat from life. One twentieth-century style of retreat has shown itself most vividly in the arts, a phenomenon that has been admirably described by Peter Abbs.[3] The practice and theory of art, Abbs maintains, has become alienated from its intrinsic nature. The primary aesthetic experience is no longer of central importance and has been usurped by non-artistic factors. In particular, there is a denial of tradition and a craving for innovation. What is new is what is good, the model for this belief being science and technology. People respond to art discursively rather than aesthetically.

The implication of Pop Art was that:

These things are real for contemporary society, therefore they should be the real objects in art! Hence, the sheep in formaldehyde. This movement, labelled Modernism, inevitably led to a collapse of imagination and a state of exhaustion. But how should we assess what followed? Is Postmodernism any truer to the aesthetic? Certainly it did not ignore the past, but its relationship with the past lacked continuity and coherence.[4]

This retreat from any faith in goodness or truth (a conception propagated by post-structural literary theory) took the form of an eclectic, detached irony:

Postmodernism tethers the power of passion and makes neutral all values, casting all creation into the single mould of irony and cleverness. The angels it favours are angels of pantomime, light, smiling, ornamental, plastic, they are not the compelling angels of Giotto, Rilke or Cecil Collins; they do not begin to possess their transcendent gravity or their promise of ineffable possibility. Free from moral and metaphysical commitment, wedded only to parodic imagination, Postmodernism hovers like a transient rainbow over the abyss. And like a rainbow, it cannot last.[5]

Louis Sass, in his book *Madness and modernism* comes to rather similar conclusions to Abbs, extending the argument into the field of psychiatry in noting the remarkable affinities between modern art and schizophrenia.[6],[7] His comments on modernism and postmodernism bear a close resemblance to that of Abbs. In postmodernism:

Instead of being rejected, conventions are actually embraced and exaggerated in various forms of parody and pastiche; hence the avant-garde element, the alienation from tradition, emerges in a different way, not as an iconoclastic driving for radical innovation and originality but in the bemused and knowing irony or deadpan detachment with which conventional forms are mockingly displayed.[8]

Art no longer conveys an ethical or intellectual message or even the expression of intense inner feelings. Sass emphasizes the fragmentation of personality and the loss of significant external reality:

The development in the twentieth century of what has seemed a higher sophistication about human unconsciousness has been accompanied, oddly enough, by a certain fragmentation and passivation, by a loss of the self's sense of unity and of its capacity for effective or voluntary action: this has gone along with an ethic of impersonality that contrasts sharply with the romantic cult of the self.[9]

Disengagement implies a loss of a simple, direct, naïve involvement in life:

Instead of a spontaneous and naive involvement—an unquestioning acceptance of the external world, the aesthetic tradition, other human beings, and one's own feelings—both Modernism and Postmodernism are imbued with hesitation and detachment, a division or doubling in which the ego disengages from normal forms of involvement with nature and society, often taking itself, or its own experiences, as its own object.[10]

The comparable withdrawal in the field of moral philosophy is described by Julia Annas:

For although we respond to talk of cowardice and generosity, of the good life and happiness, the trend of moral thinking in the twentieth century has been such that it has been hard to take these thoughts seriously as part of moral thinking. They have remained important in everyday thinking, but most moral theories have not found room for them, and reflection on them has tended to migrate into popular psychology.[11]

To put this phenomenon in another way: twentieth-century art and culture has retreated from direct involvement in ordinary experience. In using the word 'ordinary' I have in mind approaches to living which enable people to manage everyday life (with whatever limited success) rather than those which rely on one special approach, or a conglomeration of discrete special approaches to achieve whatever is desired. This question has important implications for psychotherapy, but before pursuing those I would like to try to clarify a widespread confusion about the word 'ordinary'.

The dividing line between actions that are aspects of our normal competence and those which can only be adequately carried out by people with special training is not sharply definable. In our society it is considered normal to be able to drive a car—but we have to be trained to do it and provide evidence of competence. We do not, as yet, have to prove competence in bringing up children, despite the fact that it is an incomparably more difficult task than driving a car: child-rearing, like making love or getting married, remains in the realm of the ordinary. Yet, increasingly, what is considered a matter of expertise—and, thereby a means of achieving status in a special field—encroaches on our everyday life. On one occasion, when a patient was disparaging the man-in-the-street to me, I commented that I myself was a 'man-in-the-street'. 'Oh no!', she quickly exclaimed, 'you're a professional!'.

In *The Times*, George Walden, in an article on the Booker Prize, wrote:

Usually we are called upon to applaud everything indiscriminately, and to ask no questions. In this sense the British live under a kind of benign, democrative tyranny: the tyranny of ordinariness. The victims of course, are ordinary, intelligent people who are encouraged to aspire, at the most, to the mediocre.[12]

The juxtaposition of the word 'ordinary' in consecutive sentences aptly demonstrates our ambiguity in the use of the word. In the former sentence it is clearly equated with—and denigrated by—the concept 'mediocre'. In the latter sentence, however, the people described as 'ordinary' are said to be intelligent and there are no overtones of inferiority: they are ordinary in the sense of constructing their lives in ways which do not happen to include specializing in the writing of novels or literary criticism. Yet, can we be sure that Walden, if only unconsciously, is not comparing them unfavourably with those who are gifted (or at least proficient) in these arts? Why does he not notice the discrepancy in his two uses of the word? This occurrence is no chance: we are not dealing with a minor matter of terminology but a fundamental confusion of a major concept of living. We are confronted with the question as to how we attribute value to human beings.

The term 'ordinary', as I am using it, is expressed by Doris Lessing who writes, in recalling her experience of giving birth:

Again and again, in reminiscences, novels, autobiographies, one reads of how white people have been given ordinary, decent human warmth by black people when they needed it.[13]

There is no ambiguity here. The term is used to applaud a quality to be found in people who, in this particular writer's experience, are almost invariably deemed inferior.

Those whose experience of life is bereft of meaning or is constituted by overwhelming feelings of shame will eschew the state of ordinariness. Instead, they will be inclined either to search for a meaningful life in terms of an artificially cultivated excitement or will seek a status which raises them above the common herd: they may claim special gifts, special connections, or, in the bureaucratic society in which we live, they may become experts. Moreover, not only are we in an age of experts, we are in an age of observers—not the simple, direct regard of life but the processing of experience into more manageable form; we not only search, we research; we monitor and quantify to a degree that impoverishes and distorts the experience itself. We turn back on ourselves, suffering a heightened self-consciousness.

There are several ways in which psychotherapy has been afflicted by this contemporary malaise. In an age of experts we seek an expert in living. But the nature of the particular expertise claimed by the therapist is not clear. Whereas, for example, the physician can demonstrate areas in which he possesses effective technical skills, in the case of psychotherapy we cannot be so sure. We do not really know how the undertaking works and there are numerous different techniques which are claimed to be effective in alleviating the same affliction. A profusion of research projects produce conflicting results and there is marked disagreement about the desired aim of therapy. Yet, if the profession is to have any justification for its existence, it would seem necessary for it to be able to demonstrate that its practitioners possess a competence beyond that obtained in the ordinary course of living. In the face of this dilemma the temptation to emphasize the value of a special way of behaving towards patients and a special theory and language to explain this behaviour is overwhelming. Moreover, as in the field of art, there is enormous pressure to produce ever-new techniques: the latest is the best. And Babel has arrived.

Also, psychotherapy, by its very nature, involves the practitioner in standing back to take a look at the problem—a second look, for the first look by the patient has failed. The therapist cannot simply enjoy regarding and relating to the other person as she might do in everyday life; there is a job to be done; many of those who seek help are in a state of crisis—something has gone wrong and the therapist needs to take a look at this, just as the motorist whose car breaks down mid-journey needs to look at (or get someone else to look at) the workings of the machine. However, when we have to stop and consider a problem we do not thereby stop ordinary living. Ordinary living consists (much more than many of us would choose to be the case) of problems that have to be examined. The fact that what is being looked at in psychotherapy is a person complicates matters but does not put the phenomenon into another realm of being: there are still two people in the room, living together, making the best (or worst) of it during their time together, and in their struggles to make a go of things as fellows on this planet. The importance of standing back in psychotherapy can easily be exaggerated. If we do not, in our present ignorance, know what kind of relationship is of most benefit to those in distress, then we are unjustified in making the assumption (so widespread in psychotherapy) that deeply considered reflection is necessarily the correct approach. And we should take note of the fact that excessive restraint in most intimate relationships results in emotional impoverishment on both sides. Any psychotherapeutic endeavour that relies on a technique is vulnerable to this kind of failure, including the practice of all those, like myself, who have learned their trade in the Freudian school and who value what they have learnt.

Indeed, psychoanalysis, and its varieties, have vulnerabilities all of their own.

Psychoanalysis claims to have access to an area so far removed from our ordinary experience that it requires a long and difficult training to learn how to explore this realm and a long and difficult task for the man-in-the-street to make use of the treatment and gain experience of this area; in other words, it is a very special accomplishment. Moreover, as Gellner argues, the Freudian unconscious is a very seductive concept (a 'cunning broker'), which inspires awe because it is not only a theoretical system but a social programme and points the way to a unique salvation. 'He who can guide the sufferer along the path, is automatically vindicated in his authority and standing.'[14]

Gellner maintains that psychoanalysis is sufficiently rooted in ordinary life—in our biological heritage and our capacity to make meaning of human existence—to claim our respect as a pragmatic measure to combat our confusions and pains yet requires us to submit to an extraordinarily abstract theory and practice in order to benefit. What we need to question is first, whether in order to make use of Freud's insights, we need to go through the particular hoop he improvised for that purpose, and secondly, whether his insights, however rewarding, justify a degree of specialization that inevitably omits many of the myriad ways in which one person may hope to help the emotional distress of another. The fact that a psychotherapist's technique may have, in part, been engendered by a denigration of more ordinary competencies does not necessarily mean that it is useless; but it does mean that we should look at it with a great deal of circumspection and not be so dazzled that we neglect more obvious and well-tried measures for bringing relief to anguish. In short, the paradigm of psychotherapeutic endeavour is skewed by a retreat from the ordinary, and we need to explore some of the everyday ways of being and thinking that may be of more value in the work than any method, but are prevented from coming to fruition if method is the hallmark of the work.

To what extent do therapists believe what their patients say, and is the degree of their trust in patients' statements different from that in everyday living? In ordinary life, we make our judgements of the truth of statements primarily on the basis of our knowledge of the person and the context of his speech. We may have a characteristic tendency either towards naïvety on the one hand or scepticism on the other, but it is unusual for people to discount the particular source and circumstances and content of the statement which make it seem likely to be true or false. There are, however, cultural trends of thought, which lead in one direction or the other. Freud's work has inclined us towards doubting the authenticity of statements. People, we realize, are not only disposed to purposely dissemble but do so without recognizing that they are doing it. Despite the fact, however, that the 'Freudian slip' has become part of our intellectual heritage, we do not, on the whole, go around looking for such slips; we behave to each other, in relation to the matter of truthful statements, much as we have always done.

In the psychotherapist's consulting room the patient's words are not so readily taken on trust. There are several reasons for this. First, any therapist who has been influenced by Freud will be more likely than most to expect people to indulge in unconscious denial of the truth. Secondly, to the extent that the therapeutic encounter fosters transference from the patient's experience of parents during childhood, the patient will be in a state of illusion; the qualities he perceives in the therapist are readily considered to be mere projections. Thirdly, statements by patients are often painful to the therapist, especially those which constitute an aggressive attack. In the interests of self-protection it is useful for the therapist to distance herself from them—to disbelieve them, or at least fail to give them the benefit of the doubt ('It is not I who am dogmatic, it is his father'). There is a danger that she may use this measure in order to avoid recognizing her own limitations.

Fourthly, there is a secondary gain in the enjoyment of the puzzle. This is not only the challenge of trying to help someone but the fascination of solving an enigma: what is going on below the surface? What else can the patient mean? The temptation to demonstrate shrewdness is similar to that which can afflict a writer or speaker who likes to shock, to be paradoxical and gnomic: '*You* may, in your naïvety, assume that you really think this, but I'll surprise you' (this is not to say that shocks, when appropriate, cannot be electrifyingly effective).

It may be useful at this point to consider the influence of postmodern thought on the question of psychoanalytic interpretation. One of the first analysts to take cognizance of this movement was Donald Spence,[15] who challenges the orthodox Freudian view that interpretations can lead us to historical truth. By contrast, he believes that the pressure on patient and analyst to make sense—to provide a coherent narrative—is so great that what is agreed upon is no more than a satisfying gloss. The search for meaning, he maintains, is especially insidious because it succeeds.

Spence's argument reinforces the view, outlined above, that enthusiastic adoption of Freud's method to uncover the unconscious may easily lead us away from the truths apparent to the man-in-the-street. One would therefore expect Spence to suggest that the psychoanalyst approach her task with greater humility than is the custom, look more into the degree to which she projects her theories on to the patient and note the advantages of a more ordinary dialogue. But not a bit of it. Spence assures us that analyst and patient telling each other untrue stories need not worry us at all, that if they give a narrative coherence to a life that appeared to the patient to be random or chaotic then she can feel she has done a good job.

There is some appeal in this line of thought. It helps us to escape from the narrowness of the early scientific model of psychoanalysis and brings us more into the present; it lays emphasis on the imaginative role of the therapist; on her ability, like that of the artist, to stimulate new thoughts and feelings and create rather than recreate; and it reminds us that there are many valid ways of expressing a truth other than the contemporary positivistic one. Nevertheless, Spence's view of psychoanalysis is misguided and dangerous. Useful interpretations, he believes—those he refers to as 'formal'—clothe an anomalous happening in 'respectability and take away some of its strangeness and mystery'. The task of the analyst is to search for formal—usually linguistic—similarities between the experience to be investigated and other features in the patient's life. By means of such linking a new and convincing *gestalt* can be made and the patient is comforted.

However, if there is no appeal to factual or emotional truth but only to formal truth then there are no means by which the analyst and patient can tell whether they are merely building up a coherent but defensive pattern—the formation of a *false self*. It is all too easy—as the propagandist so well knows—to use similarities to convince people of whatever one happens to want to convince them of; and Spence, at times, comes uncomfortably near to presenting psychoanalysis as nothing more than a form of propaganda. Indeed, there are passages in which he makes such damaging criticisms of psychoanalysis while continuing to commend it that one wonders, momentarily, whether the whole exercise is a subtle attempt to send up his colleagues. But it isn't.

Spence's hypothesis undermines a belief in the ordinary nature of therapeutic healing not, as Freud did, by emphasizing the expertise of the analyst in finding the truth but in trying to persuade us that we need not, as in everyday life, concern ourselves with the truth of what people say, but can more usefully use our imaginative powers to create plausible narratives. It may well be that the therapist who works in this way may be more successful, as is the artist, if he can produce a narrative which is true to human nature, but he does not feel the need to dirty his fingers in messy details of factual truth. I will give an example of an interchange which seemed to me to be no more suffused with illusion than conversations in daily life, yet arguably no less a part of a therapeutic endeavour than much that we do in therapy.

A woman was expressing dismay at the (supposed) fact that she had few friends and was presumably disliked. We talked about this for a while, then I asked: 'Do *you* like other people?' Her answer was, 'I don't know what to say. My mind's gone blank.' There was a silence, broken by her asking me: 'What are you thinking?' I reflected and told her my thoughts as honestly as I could. 'I'm having two thoughts. Firstly, I've got a twitch at this moment from my tooth which has an abscess and I'm worried I might lose it. Secondly, I'm wondering whether you would care about my abscess if I told you.'

The patient was taken aback. We were no longer having a dispassionate discussion; we were now in an interpersonal, emotional, everyday confrontation. At first she was angry. She felt that my question had undermined any spontaneous response she might have had and that I was trying to make her feel guilty in the way that so many people seemed to have done in her life. But it also caused her to think in a concrete way about the matter that had previously made her mind blank. And this, I think, was useful.

At this point in the session we were not, I feel sure, telling each other stories. I think my answer was as true as I could reasonably hope to get. My tooth was hurting, I had become aware of this, and I did wonder what her reaction to my discomfort and anxiety might be. I mention this exchange for two reasons. First, as a simple example of the fact that contact with reality is not, or need not, be lost just because two people are engaged in a process that we call therapy; secondly, that the confrontation of a true fact in therapy can be useful. It may seem a bit absurd for me to stress such an obvious point, but I do so as a countermeasure to scepticism over the possibility of analytical psychotherapy being anything other than the exchange of illusions, guesswork, imagination, and rhetoric.

When someone is motivated by the urge to gain relief from emotional anguish we are likely to feel sympathetic and encouraged to make the effort required to help despite resistance to our attempts. Less easy to approach are those who possess characteristics which jar on us, make us uneasy, yet are difficult to formulate. Often, such qualities are manifestations of narcissism: behaviour which derives from an attempt to preserve the self at the expense of others.

In the example I quote I did no more than express my doubts about the patient's capacity to care spontaneously about people. This was not easy to express, not because I feared her vulnerability (which is often the reason to avoid such a comment) but because her narcissism was so elusive, and I expected and feared an angry and defensive retaliation, which would be likely to include a comment on my own self-interest and lack of professionalism. Donna is, in most ways, an admirable person; a loving and responsible mother and a dedicated and capable social worker with a keen sense of justice. Yet on this occasion, because I sometimes felt the need (which happened to coincide with her request for a truthful statement) to pursue my impression that, in order to preserve her poise and because of certain disappointments in life she withheld her consideration of others, including me. However, although I am deeply influenced by Freud it could be said with justification that what I described is hardly a psychoanalytic interpretation—indeed, it might well be thought a technical error to respond so simply. How, then, when considering the place of truth in therapy, are we to conceive a more typically psychoanalytic response? In an orthodox analytic setting the therapist would be unlikely to respond directly to the patient's question: 'What are you thinking?' and would, indeed, see her role as one in which the *patient's* pain was the only consideration.

Leaving aside the argument that such self-effacement (the 'blank screen') will enable fantasies to develop and be interpreted, it is easy to see why such a passively receptive attitude be recommended. The therapist is there to listen, understand, and help and is being paid for it, and some patients are so fragile that all their energy is directed into trying to survive. A danger, however, in a uniformly facilitating attitude is the ease with which the patient can be left with, or even encouraged towards, a complacent acceptance of their narcissism: their lack of consideration for the needs of the other person in the room can seem quite appropriate and remain unconfronted and unseen; consequently, their selfishness can remain intact. Insofar as the therapist follows Freud's directive to efface herself, she may easily lead the patient away from everyday living.

There is a further paradox. Although the stereotype of the psychoanalytic session inhibits straight talking between people, Freud did manage to get them in a room together to talk and he directed them towards looking at what was actually going on between them (in psychoanalytic terms, the 'transference' and 'countertransference'), an undertaking which, if one gets rid of the theory, leads us to something actual, immediate, and unspecialized—and, potentially, a path to truths which can be evaded by social conventions. This is one way of conceiving the interchange described above. It is, however, significant that I have had to struggle to put it in this simple way rather than resort to orthodox psychoanalytic terms such as 'countertransference'. The essential form of the verbal exchange was: she asked me what I was thinking and I told her.

The grasp of ordinary living can also be easily lost if the therapist departs too readily from immediate and near-to-hand matters, which are more accessible to truth, and speculates in areas of fantasy and remote history with a confidence that is misconceived. It is to this latter tendency that Spence's criticisms of psychoanalysis should be directed. There is nothing wrong with an attempt to come to the truth, as best one can, about matters which are far removed in place and time—indeed, quite the reverse—provided that the search is undertaken with rigour and the two people are prepared to accept that the most they can do may be no more than the best conjecture possible on the available evidence. But this is not to live in the illusion of a convenient narrative. It is no more and no less that the means we use in ordinary life whereby we establish some truths with certainty, some with a reasonable confidence, and some with no more than the most plausible explanation we can find. Ways of thinking that depart from common sense can indeed lead us fruitfully down new paths: we can learn an enormous amount from using ideas (e.g. anthropological) which come from another discipline and, in our own field, from those who work with very disturbed ('psychotic') people whom many psychotherapists confront only occasionally. But we also have to note the contradictions, aberrations, and exaggerations that are often involved in hypotheses, and use our own experience of living and working to avoid being carried too far by ideas that do not have their origin in our daily experience with others. It may be that a future generation may come to believe that individuals do not exist and that conventions have no truth content, and can live by such beliefs: but, as we are now, we cannot bridge the gap between such ideas and our actual experience of living. We are best served by relying, as therapists, on those conceptions that enable us to get through the day. It is surprising how often a valuable critique of orthodox thinking is rendered harmful by overstating the case. If Spence had been satisfied in showing the limitations of psychoanalytic interpretation, he would have done a service to the profession and brought us nearer to a realistic appraisal of reality.

One unhappy effect of the postmodernist's savage dismantling of our confidence in our perceptions is the tendency of some thinkers to take the matter of therapy less seriously. This, I believe, is the case with Adam Phillips, who urges us to find psychoanalysis 'interesting' rather than 'important'. It is a worthy undertaking to attack, as Phillips does with style in his book *Terrors and experts*,[16] the pompousness and solemnity of a profession which overestimates its expertise; it is another to approach the work with ironic detachment. Paradoxically, although Freud is considered, as a man of the Enlightenment, to be far removed from postmodernism—indeed, Phillips makes much of this distinction—there is perhaps a closer connection than is usually recognized. What is happening in the room is not considered by the analyst to be quite real. It is rather akin to theatre. The patient's words, although listened to with the utmost care, are not regarded as communications which require the kind of response that would be considered appropriate in ordinary life. They are not, in a sense, taken seriously. What I am trying to identify is a *pervasive* attitude of detachment. An appropriate response in everyday living to a particular communication may well be irony, humour, or play; lack of such responses results, indeed, in an impoverished withdrawal from much that is good in life. The question is whether the analyst (postmodernist or not) manages to create an atmosphere that goes beyond mere role-playing and gives the possibility of intimacy. Psychotherapy is nothing if not important and intimate. My heart has often sunk when I have made a comment to a patient and he has responded by saying: 'How interesting!'

How does one convey the difference between 'important' and 'self-important'? How does one describe intimacy? In writing above about the importance of psychotherapy and the importance of bringing reality and intimacy into the consulting room I feel embarrassed. What I have written seems stilted and pompous. Quite apart from my own personal limitations it is perhaps inevitable that a therapist can hardly hope to describe, without seeming presumptuous, significant experiences in therapy. Not being a poet, I can no more do so effectively than I could convey the occasional (and all too rare) feelings of transcendence when I see something beautiful or poignant. Approaching the question indirectly lets me describe something that happened recently.

A therapist came to me for supervision. She is experienced and extremely effective. Instead of talking about a patient, as she usually does, she told me of the feeling of anxiety that had overtaken her on coming back to work after a brief holiday. 'I felt quite at a loss,' she said, 'and I thought: What is this about? What am I doing? Can I do it? Should I be a therapist at all?'

She was quite serious about this. I was puzzled, for I refer patients to her with the utmost confidence; yet not puzzled, for, as I admitted to her, I often feel somewhat similar. During our discussion she regretted the fact that she had no certain theoretical framework to guide her, a fact which did not surprise me in someone who works so intuitively. 'I suppose I can only rely,' she said, 'on whether it feels all right or not, and just talking about it, as I'm doing with you. But sometimes I feel it's just not good enough to work this way. I ought to be able to formulate it—and that doubt often spoils it for me.' It seemed that the therapist was working very well, probably in a quite gifted way, but that her enjoyment with clients was marred by an inability to express her experience in discursive prose. She could not believe (for there is no theory to validate it) that her intuition, passion, spontaneity, and enjoyment were aspects of her therapeutic competence. (A man once said to me: 'The most important thing a therapist can do for me is to enjoy me'.) For better or worse it is perhaps those of us with less humility who attempt to convey such experiences in words.

Recently, I damaged my hand on a rose thorn. As the cut was rather deep I took myself off to the accident room of the main hospital. I was treated, by the doctor and nurse, with courtesy, kindness, and warmth. I did not feel that they were acting according to some formulation about doctor/patient or nurse/patient relationships. It seemed to me that they were doing something that they liked doing, took a pride in doing, and were allowing their ordinary decency to have its say. (I am quite aware of the horrors of understaffing and unacceptable waiting lists and I know that this kind of friendly caring does not always occur in the profession of medicine and nursing, but I think it occurs far more often than not, and does so despite all the obstacles to ordinariness that I discuss above.) The psychotherapeutic situation has enormous advantages over a short encounter in an accident department in enabling a positive relationship to take place, but the dangers of inhibiting such a development are more subtle.

In dwelling on the forms of retreat that are characteristic of our time I do not want to forget that there are other styles, rooted in traditions that have held sway in the past and which still affect us despite their attenuated potency. I particularly have in mind the restrictive and life-denying elements in organized religion. One of Freud's dearest aims was to free us from its malign influence. But how successful was he in this endeavour? Psychoanalysis has its own dogma, is sometimes likened to a religion, and Freud's ideas have been shown to contain elements from the Judeo-Christian background of his culture.[17, 18] To what extent, for example, is the tone of earnestness, hard to define, that so often characterizes psychotherapeutic lectures or discussion a descendent—well-modified—of the priestly voice? More than once, during a seminar, a colleague has commented to me, 'I wish I didn't feel I was in church'.

It may be that because I am the child of God-fearing Presbyterian parents in a provincial town that I am oversensitive to the heaviness of a moralistic atmosphere (as well as being conditioned by it) but I know from what others tell me that I am not alone in this susceptibility. In reference to psychotherapy it is often caricatured by such mannerisms as the knowing grunts and 'ah-ha's of the imagined therapist. Insofar as this judgement holds some truth, it serves as a warning to the practitioner, for it is not only the validity of interpretation but the style of the conversation that may help to release someone from the power of his 'super-ego'. I am reminded of the first patient to arrive when I set up practice in Cambridge. I had never seen him before, but he had been referred by someone who had been in therapy with me. He said, 'Hi Pete! I hear you need patients so I'm volunteering.' Do I analyse his defences, do I say 'Ah-ha', do I give a wan smile, or do I respond in kind?

Films by Ingmar Bergman give a formidable rendering of the heaviness of our psychologically oppressive family life. By contrast, a film directed by one of his compatriots, Lasse Hallström, *My Life as a Dog*, evokes an entirely different atmosphere—although it is not without tragedy. The hero, a boy of eleven or twelve, is sent to live with his uncle. At the workplace of the uncle is a very attractive and curvaceous woman who makes friends with the boy. One day she asks him to come with her, as a kind of chaperone, to the studio of an artist who wishes to paint her in the nude. He does so, and from where he sits he can only get a tantalizing view of what is going on. During the second visit his desire to get a proper sighting of this voluptuous woman is more than he can bear. Noticing that there is a skylight above her, he creeps out on to the roof and peers through the skylight. Inevitably, given his frantic excitement, he crashes through to the floor.

The next scene shows the boy sitting on a bench, with a fair number of minor cuts, but basically unharmed. The woman has her arm round him. I wish I could describe the expression on her face: she is smiling, amused, flattered, loving, mischievous, compassionate.

> 'Did you see anything?' she asks.
> He looks at her solemnly, 'I saw *everything*', he answers.
> 'You won't get confirmed you know, if you do this sort of thing.'
> There is a pause. 'It was worth it,' he says.
> She gives him a hug.

As I watched this film I found myself yearning for an experience I had too little of as a child: that someone would bring that kind of lightheartedness—not irresponsible, not prurient—to sexuality and other matters. It seemed like a breath of God's fresh air in a musty confined space. What word should one use for such an experience? I cannot find one: the best I can do is 'ordinary' or perhaps 'straightforward'—a quality that involves lightness and flexibility, that does not stifle with dogma and rigid principle, and must not itself be elevated to a dogma. But how to achieve this lightness? And, if we do achieve it, how on earth to convey it?

To give prominence to the concept of ordinariness in psychotherapy is, I know from experience, to lay oneself open to many kinds of criticism. It is impossible to define the word with any degree of precision or in a way that would meet with general acceptance: it is all things to all men. It can be used, too easily, for defensive or pretentious purposes. When George Steiner, for example, refers to himself as an ordinary person we suspect him of false modesty. It does not have the ring of truth.

Despite those shortcomings and in lieu of a satisfactory alternative I shall continue to use the word to describe an aim and experience which I believe to be central to any mutual and intimate engagement between two people. It stands against pretensions of superiority and the loss of immediacy that occurs when a preoccupation with theory and technique take precedence. Wilfrid Bion's arresting and inspiring admonition to enter the consulting room 'without memory or desire' had something of this quality, yet, if taken literally rather than poetically, conveys a picture of an extraordinary controlled effort to act in a precise way according to a strict concept. In ordinary life we do well to focus our attention on the other person, free from distraction, prejudice, and preconception, but we do not strain towards an extreme state of mind, and it would be distancing to do so.

It is the sanity of ordinary living that is perhaps its most valuable asset. The capacity of the man-in-the-street to find humour in situations of fear and turmoil or his ability to see through cant keeps the show on the road. It is not to be confused with conventionality; the child who says of the Emperor: 'Look, he has no clothes!' is, to my mind, being ordinary. Of course, it doesn't always work; but nothing comes with a guarantee. And when we seek, in law, a final judgement on the acts of our fellow men and women, we turn to the ordinary person. It is for similar reasons, I believe, that when, as therapists, we are lost, the thought: 'What would I believe best in such a case in my ordinary life?' is not a thought to be readily dismissed.

I will end with a description of an interchange, made available to me by my friend Vicki Gardiner, who is a Jungian analyst.

During my Christmas break from patients I had determined to be more analytically on the ball when sessions recommenced in the New Year. I had spent some time reviewing my work during the break and had decided that I was missing too many valuable opportunities for analysis of patients' material. Shortly after resuming consultations and bearing in mind my resolution, a postcard arrived from a woman patient who had been working with me a number of years. The subject of this was Botticelli's "The return of Judith" and depicted two women, one of whom carried the decapitated head of a man. The content of her written message was obscure and I decided I should re-present it to her for our joint exploration as to the possible meaning. She was very resistant to this idea and insisted that the card did not in any way convey angry feelings towards me or the process we were involved in together.

At our next meeting she arrived flushed and agitated. Hardly inside the consulting room, she insisted that I should remain silent whilst she said what needed saying. I have to say I was stunned into silence as this previously very obedient patient unleashed what seemed to be the suppressed fury of a lifetime. She told me that she was sick of my interpretations and thoughts and no longer wanted to consider either. She went on through her rage and her tears and when finally her passion seemed spent she lifted her head to look directly at me and with enormous longing said: 'Don't you see I just want you to be my friend?'

References

1. Asan, E. (1999). The limits of technique in family therapy. In *Committed uncertainty: Essays in honour of Peter Lomas*. (ed. L. King), p. 120. Whurr, London.
2. Smail, D. (1996). *How to survive without psychotherapy*, p. 204. Constable, London.
3. Abbs, P. (1996). *The politics of imagination*. Skool Books, London.
4. Ibid., p. 7.
5. Ibid., p. 22.
6. Sass, L. (1992). *Madness and modernism. Insanity in the light of modern art, literature and thought*. Harvard University Press, Cambridge, MA.
7. Sass, L. (1995). *The paradoxes of delusion: Wittgenstein, Schreber and the schizophrenic mind*. Cornell University Press, Ithaca, NY.
8. Ibid., p. 30.
9. Ibid., p. 7.
10. Ibid., p. 37.
11. Annas, J. (1993). *The morality of happiness*, p. 10. Oxford University Press.
12. Walden, G. (1995). *The Times*, 8 November.
13. Lessing, D. (1994). *Under my skin*, p. 218. HarperCollins, London.
14. Gellner, E. (1985). *The psychoanalytic movement*. Paladin, London.
15. Spence, D. (1984). *Narrative truth and historical truth*. Norton, New York.
16. Phillips, A. (1995). *Terrors and experts*. Faber, London.
17. Rieff, P. (1965). *The mind of the moralist*. Methuen, London.
18. Webster, R. (1995). *Why Freud was wrong*. HarperCollins, London.

3

The myth of neutrality

Moral philosophers cannot avoid taking sides, and would-be neutral philosophers merely take sides surreptitiously.

Iris Murdoch

In his critique of contemporary psychiatry, David Ingleby writes:

The traditional objection to bringing values into scientific debate is, of course, that the argument then collapses into a relativistic free-for-all which is the very antithesis of what science is supposed to be. However, Kuhn's close examination of the history of science showed that the grounds on which one paradigm is preferred to another are not exclusively scientific ones: the determinants of that choice lie to a large extent outside science, in social and psychological factors . . . This view has naturally been hotly contested, since it blurs almost to vanishing-point the distinction between scientific belief-systems and (say) religious or political ones; but . . . Kuhn's conclusion is only disastrous if one presupposes, as he and most scientists traditionally have, that any choice determined by social or psychological factors is necessarily an irrational one.[1]

Psychotherapists, alas, are not free from the prejudice indicated by Ingleby, although one might expect them to be less impressed by the positivistic approach than their colleagues in psychiatry because the criteria for assessing their work are much less amenable to contemporary scientific method; moreover, they are forced, in their daily encounters, to enter more closely into personal dilemmas of a moral nature. Many, if not most psychotherapists do, in fact, have a notable interest in the question of how we should live. They read books by philosophers, religious leaders, and social thinkers. Some psychotherapists go into print themselves on the subject, giving their views, for example, on how to bring up children. Because those who come for help have lost their way in life it is hardly surprising that therapists should be interested in this question. The patient's loss may be profound. He or she may have entered a dark world in which all meaning has gone; they simply do not know how to survive the day and cannot even go through the motions of ordinary living. Or, in a less devastating way, they find themselves blocked in a limited area of their lives. In either case the therapist is faced with matters that confront his views on how to live.

The question which presents itself at this point is: 'How does the therapist manage to avoid confronting the fact that he is continuously embroiled in questions of morality?' One element in his denial is, I think, a confusion over what it means to know how to live. It can easily be thought of as a purely physical matter. We learn how to live in the physical world— to walk, to climb, to avoid fire, and later, we learn the technical accomplishments, like riding a bicycle, that are appropriate to our particular civilization. But as we learn the rules of the game in our society—how to speak, when to speak, what to say or do in certain situations—the ground is less solid. Does society know the best way to live? Is it a sure guide to the great or small issues with which we must perennially wrestle? Should I have long or short hair? What should I do with my life? Should I work regular hours or become a drop-out? Should I live for the present or in order to build up a secure future? Questions of this kind—questions that are enmeshed in morality—regularly make their appearance in the psychotherapeutic session. And there are situations about which the patient may have no moral problem but the therapist does—for example, someone who is HIV positive and is taking risks with the lives of others.

Let me take an extreme, and hypothetical, example. If the patient does not see an elephant in the room because there is none there, the therapist makes no comment. If however, another patient, in similar circumstances, reports seeing an elephant the therapist pricks up his ears, observes a mistaken perception, and speaks accordingly. In a much less obvious way the same dynamic occurs in the moral sphere. If the patient sees a moral situation in the same way as does the therapist there is unlikely to be an exploration of it. If, however, he says or does something which, in the eyes of the therapist, is morally wrong or is a sign of moral blindness ('I think cripples are offensive to the eye and should not be allowed in public places'), then he will feel a criticism that may or may not lead to an immediate confrontation but which will be noted for future consideration. It is only because, as mentioned earlier, we do not tend to take the moral world as real in the way we regard the physical world that the two cases (the physical and the moral) are taken to be quite distinct and have nothing in common. The fact that there is much more likelihood of agreement over physical matters than moral ones does not mean that differences of opinion may not, in both cases, require comparable debate. I will now give a few examples of sessions which are in no way out of the ordinary and in which moral questions arise.

A woman arrived in a fury. She had taken her children to hospital for a routine check. The hospital car park was overflowing. Eventually she found a space and was backing in to it when a car quickly came along and nipped in before her. As the man got out she said: 'Didn't you see I was here first?'. 'I've a clinic to run,' said the man, without apology, and walked off. She was furious.

The patient then went for her appointment, waited several hours, and observed with amazement the resigned patience of those who had been kept waiting. Again she was furious, and felt like complaining. 'This kind of resignation wouldn't happen,' she said, 'in X' (her country of origin).

How should the therapist respond to this account? I could have interpreted that her rage was a transference from her father, who she had felt was not there for her. Or that it was a displacement from a transference to me who, in a sense, keeps her waiting for something she wants but never gets. On the other hand, was her anger appropriate? Where do I stand on the deficiencies of the health service, on medical arrogance, or on the merits of patience? Was the consultant justified or not in seizing the car space and dashing off? Is it right or wrong to accept with patience the understaffing and long queues of the health service? What I think on these issues will colour my response to her.

Another patient, Rachel, told me how angry she felt that her husband gave so much money to his parents. 'He's very generous,' she said. 'He's continually giving money to them. But I resent it. How are we going to pay for holidays and the children's schooling? Am I mean? Am I greedy?'

I asked Rachel if she had confronted her husband about the matter. 'No,' she said, 'I think he knows I resent it, but I feel I have no right to. He earns the money; the money is his.'

I said that this was a debatable question, that nowadays many people, particularly those women influenced by feminism, would question the husband's right to do what he liked with the money, however good his motives and however generous he was towards her. 'I know they would,' she said, 'But I don't feel that way. What you say gives me a sinking feeling in my stomach. It makes me think of when my stepmother took away all my pocket-money for herself and I couldn't do anything about it. I had no rights at all. My father just didn't care what happened.'

It seems likely that the childhood impingement and her present passivity in the face of what might be considered unjustified were related. Rachel had come to the interpretation herself. But what had made that particular interpretation possible was influenced by my own moral view on husband–wife relationships and the observation I made in the light of it.

James came to me because he felt quite lost in life and unable to make decisions. He had done well in the academic world and achieved a good university post, but found that his desire to continue with his job had quite faded. Indeed, it seemed that he had never had a great enthusiasm for the work and it was remarkable that, despite a lack of inner commitment, he had achieved this position. In the consulting room he expressed himself in a very physical way: he had mobile features, a ready laugh, and gesticulated as he conversed. At times I found myself imagining that he would be more at home with a rope around his waist, climbing the north face of the Eiger.

During the course of our discussions James spoke of his pleasure in using his hands and of the enjoyment he got from the feel of the natural things of the world—pebbles, for example. 'I feel trapped,' he said. 'Trapped in my work, trapped in everything. I'd be better in a Mediterranean country or in South America, where the pace is slower.' These occasional exclamations, however, were not made with any conviction. Most of the time (when we were not discussing his childhood or his relation with me) he agonized over his wish to hold his present life together in a way that would please those around him, and felt quite inadequate to the task. The thoughts that occurred to me were as follows:

1. For some reason James had grown up feeling a misfit and had chosen to put the requirements of the world before his own natural inclinations. (In psychoanalytical terms he had repressed his instincts or buried his 'true self'.) We needed to explore why and how this had happened.
2. The only way forward I could envisage that would reduce his anguish would be for him to follow his inclinations more: yet these seemed to fly in the face of economic reality and his love of and responsibility towards his family.
3. His indictment of contemporary society as a frenetic rush, corrupting to the soul, was one which many people would endorse.

We were enmeshed in the question not only: 'How should *he* live best?', but: 'What sort of life, in general terms, is a good one to live and in what ways does society act against this'. I do not know what I would have advised myself to do in comparable circumstances. To pretend, however, that there was no present moral dilemma, or that I had no views on living which had any bearing on the subject would, I believe, have been absurd and hypocritical.

These examples are about specific problems. I will now return to Rachel, who I mentioned earlier, and give an account of an interchange in which our general views on life did not emerge from a particular predicament. Rachel told me the following dream:

My sister had become a member of the Merovingians. I was there too and there were a lot of people wandering through the woods and fields. I like it and feel at home amongst these people, but there was no water and this troubled me. A man who was a member of the group said: "I'm lonely because Christ is dead and I'm without him."

I thought: "Yes, I can understand that he would feel lonely without him."

Rachel then told me what she knew about the Merovingians who had been a powerful force in Southern France and had strange beliefs—that, for instance, Christ had not died on the cross but had fled to France and that some of his ancestors were living there now.

I've always had a thing about Christ or, rather, what he stood for. I don't go to church, or read the bible, or pray, but he means something special to me. When I was young I had some overwhelming experience at communion—you'll think me mad—they felt quite weird, everything seemed to come together in the world and I felt embraced and abandoned myself.

Rachel has often expressed distrust of evangelical groups which, she feels, take one away from reality; some committed believers, she thinks, live inside their heads, rather than in the outside world. My own impression of Rachel (and this is what she believes herself) is of a very down-to-earth person who is spontaneous and engages closely and intuitively with others.

I said that I thought that there was something in her that yearned for the certainty of a creed that would make her feel safe and that, despite her spontaneous way of being, she could be very attracted by systems of thought which purported to explain life; that, in other words, she was not completely different from those evangelic groups which she criticized.

We discussed whether this attachment was a neurotic search for an ideal. During the course of our conversation I confessed that I could very easily empathize with her transcendental feelings and that I had experienced them myself, especially when I was younger.

> Myself:—'They were just as you describe them; absolutely overwhelming and inexplicable.'
> *Rachel*:   'Yes, they feel mystical.'

I said that I seemed to have nothing to say to her about them.

> *Myself*:   'As I can't explain my own experience, I can't explain yours. But with me they were not connected with Christ.'
> *Rachel*:   'Perhaps we all find ways of articulating them as best we can. But I know Christ is central to me. I can't explain it.'

At this point Rachel was moved to tears. After a while I said, 'I realize now that I do have a line on them. For me, it is always when I'm outside, and usually when it is quiet and beautiful. I think I believe it's something to do with nature. We've lost touch with it today. It's never quiet and I think we can't get the feelings that "primitive" people got in the past.'

Rachel then said that she too experienced these feelings sometimes when walking home, alone, at night: 'There are no street lamps where I live.'

The discussion had moved away from the question of neurotic defences. I cannot be sure that experiences of this kind are not defensive but at this moment we were talking about something which we both believe to be an element of existence, and that, although we could only flounder in our attempt to express and understand it, we would not readily be prepared to explain this feeling of awe and wonder in terms other than itself. We were talking about one avenue to the appreciation of living—and perhaps recognizing experiences that have been largely lost. 'There is something wrong,' said Rachel at one point, 'in the grey faces of so many of the people I see.'

After the session I felt appalled at how little I had explored the details of the dream, particularly the meaning to her of the Merovingians. But we could always return to the dream and, indeed, did so.

I have myself had two Freudian analyses. Both of my analysts were dedicated, compassionate, and gifted interpreters and I have reason to be grateful for the insight they gave me. The first was rigidly orthodox in her technique and told me nothing about herself directly: the second was much more open but still subscribed to the ideal of neutrality. However, when I look back to that time I am in no doubt about where each of them stood on important issues about living. I learnt this from the content of their interpretations, the nuance of their tone of voice or the way they worded their questions ('Are you really working as a *navvy*?', asked my first analyst in bewilderment and distaste at one point); and occasionally, I learnt it from their direct statements. Sometimes their views on life influenced me for good; sometimes not. But in no way were they morally neutral. I have no reason to suppose that these two respected and responsible practitioners were exceptional cases.

When we are engrossed in a detective novel our focus is primarily on puzzling out the clues and piecing them together. The delight of the book is the challenge which engrosses us. Therapy, by contrast, is a serious matter and I do not want to make a flippant comparison, but we can be similarly gripped, as therapists, in the pursuit of clues, desperately anxious to make sense of what it all means, and grateful to Freud for his insights. In such a frame of mind it is understandable that we might easily forget the moral dimension of the undertaking. Our perception of Freud's neutral way of working adds greatly to this belief. But how true is this impression? Roazen reports that, while interviewing Erich Fromm, his wife was also present and:

Wondered aloud where on earth the New York analysts had gotten their technique from, since the aim of neutrality and distance seemed so foreign to how Freud himself had proceeded. Her question was an excellent one, which I have thought about a lot. I concluded later that the Americans had come to Vienna in Freud's sick phase, or identified with the relatively distant, detached, dying Freud. But there was also hypocritical disguising of what Freud had actually been like, and this shared secret became a powerful bond among Freud's loyal disciples.[2]

It is not surprising that Freud did not act with the neutrality that is attributed to him. He was a deeply moral man concerned with the basic issues of how to live. He was also moral in the colloquial sense of the word, that is, his beliefs of good conduct focused on rectitude, self-restriction, hard work, and intellectual rigour at the expense of easy, impulsive, short-term satisfaction—attributes he thought characteristic of children, and to an extent, women. Like Plato, he conceived morality in terms of conflict: the easy, thoughtless pursuit of pleasure must be mastered by informed and circumspect reason about the way to live: the right attitude is to recognize the severe limits to all our aims and wishes and to accept, without resentment, the harshness of life.

Philip Rieff, in his brilliant, if somewhat rambling, study of Freud[3] has shown that there are remarkable paradoxes in Freud's position. Although, temperamentally and intellectually, Freud favoured abstention and discipline, his theory and practice are notable for the attempt to relieve patients from the grip of a tyrannical conscience and thereby reduce the burden of their inhibitions and guilt. There is a marked conflict between the fact that Freud's work focused so much on moral dilemmas and his almost desperate desire to present psychoanalysis as a scientific and moral-free undertaking. This paradox has been the source of an immeasurable confusion and is still with us. It accounts, I think, for the fact that the work of Rieff and others who have demonstrated the moral attitudes inherent in Freudian theory has been both recognized as respectable scholarship yet largely ignored. Although Freud's instinct theory undermines any attempt to conceive the child as a moral agent responsible for his or her own decisions, his stance is set firmly in the Judaeo-Christian tradition. The child is born wicked either because he is possessed by the Devil or because this is his natural state (what might now be called his 'selfish' genes). Parents and society must prevail upon him if he is to behave well. The means for this change may be punishment, threatened punishment, reasoning, psychoanalytic insights, or an awareness of and surrender to the love of God.

In a well-argued discussion Brunner[4] reveals the degree to which Freud's theories are suffused with images and ideals of hierarchy and control. His élitist political views are mirrored in his psychological theories:

He extolled the virtues of control and warned of the dangers of balance and equality, which he associated with a weakness or even a breakdown of the mind's government, while he depicted health as based on an enlightened but élitist role. Yet Freud persistently rejects the idea that politics or morals have a bearing on his work. Analysis, he wrote, makes for *unity*, but not necessarily for *goodness*.[5]

By departing from Freud's instinct theory the 'object-relations' school of psychoanalysis made it easier to conceive of the self as a moral agent, responsible for its own actions, thus bringing it closer to the view of the man-in-the-street. It is a path that has been followed with less enthusiasm than might have been expected despite the fact that the two most influential thinkers of the object-relations school, Melanie Klein and D. W. Winnicott, in their different ways, conceived childhood development to be a moral one—a growth from self-interest to concern for others. Klein's view is that love is based on a desperate need to make reparation for destructive wishes. Salvation comes from the recognition, as experience and knowledge increases, that there is an outer world with needs of its own, and a growing capacity to take this fact into consideration. Money-Kyrle, who bases his views on Kleinian theory, is one of the earliest psychoanalysts to seriously confront the moral implications of practice.[6] The moral sense, he believes, is empirical and universal and depends on the normal development from the 'paranoid' projection of badness on to the outerworld to an acceptance of the badness within oneself. An improvement in the organization of society is of little use: changes must come from insight into one's neurotic failure of development. It is, however, debatable whether moral development consists of a gradual overcoming of an original evil. There is certainly plenty of evil around but it is, perhaps, an adultcentric point of view to emphasize this quality in the child. To do so would suggest a prejudice comparable to that of attributing evil to the so-called savages of 'primitive' society.

In a recent and wide-ranging book, Hinshelwood has elaborated the Kleinian view of moral progress by means of psychoanalysis,[7] coming out quite firmly with the statement that psychoanalysis is a moral practice. His reasoning for this opinion is that the aim of analysis is integration, and integration enhances a person's capacity for morality.

If I have understood Hinshelwood correctly he is saying that it is good to pursue a practice which helps to create the ground from which morality can flourish. In this sense psychoanalysis is certainly a moral undertaking. To my mind, however, this thesis does not confront the fact that the process by which integration is reached—interpretation—is not itself a neutral procedure free from moral bias: the analyst's aim for his patient is a much more complicated affair than simply wanting integration. Nevertheless, Hinshelwood fully recognizes, in a way that is unusual among psychoanalysts, the ease with which the practitioner may morally coerce the patient into accepting his own vision, I shall return to this theme in Chapter 9.

Neville Symington, who has been deeply influenced by both Klein's and Winnicott's theories of child development puts the case for psychoanalysis as an ethical undertaking in a somewhat different way.[8] He maintains that the basic aim of religion and psychoanalysis, at their best, are broadly the same; an attempt to free someone from his narcissism and enable him to stop deceiving himself and others:

The analysis is an ongoing battle against resistant aspects of the personality, bearing all the notes of the spiritual struggle described by mystics, both in Western and Eastern cultures.[9]

Symington writes with an attractive clarity and gives us a rich and illuminating discussion of the interconnectedness between the aims of religion and psychoanalysis recognizing that the latter constitutes a moral struggle for the patient requiring an 'inner creative emotional act'.[10] While acknowledging the importance of Jung's decisive rejection of Freud's biological orientation and his emphasis on the claims of religion, Symington is clearly exasperated by Jung's inconsistencies. The main criticism he makes is that Jung encourages the acceptance of religious dogma rather than forging one's own spiritual quest. Paradoxically, Symington himself is inconsistent in a way that is not unlike Jung. One feels he is torn between advocating a unique exploration of life and the adoption of a set of values prescribed by an established authority.

The thinkers who have confronted the moral element in psychotherapy most directly are the Existentialists. Indeed, it is to the writings of Buber, Tillich, Binswanger, and others of similar orientation that I owe much of my recognition that psychotherapy cannot be justified in terms of scientific principles. What is regrettable in the Existential school of thought, however, is the degree to which it is preoccupied with obscure philosophical argument. The flight from the ordinary is very pervasive. It appears that if we eschew religious dogma we fall into the hands of science, and if we escape from science we become dazzled by the intricacies of philosophical debate.

One of the most encouraging features of the recent psychoanalytic scene is the rehabilitation (if only partial) of Sandor Ferenczi. I sometimes think that those of us who, today, try to articulate the 'personal',[11] or 'intersubjective'[12] approach to psychotherapy have not got much further than Ferenczi's simple diary note, written in 1932:

As finally one begins to wonder whether it would not be natural and also more to the purpose to be openly a human being with feelings, empathic at times and frankly exasperated at other times.[13]

In view of the increasing awareness of the mutuality of the therapeutic relationship and the appreciation of several thinkers—some of whose work I discussed above—that therapy has a moral aim it is surprising that the myth that the practitioner is morally neutral in his actual day-to-day work remains so persistent: the moral beliefs that pervade what the therapist does and says (or avoids doing and saying) are relatively unexplored. Considerations of ethics in psychotherapy tend to focus on issues of the kind comparable to those that concern the medical profession: that is to say, on events outside the consulting room or gross misconduct within it. These include the matter of confidentiality or the relatively unusual case (an example of which would be sexual seduction by the therapist) and the problems of the profession as a whole, including a code of ethics and the availability of psychotherapy for those who need it but cannot pay private fees. It is areas such as these that are covered by Holmes and Lindley's excellent book *The values of psychotherapy*.[14]

A closer study of mutual values inside the consulting room, presents difficult questions but can also accrue benefits. One of these would be to demystify certain aspects of the therapeutic alliance. We know, from the work of Gregory Bateson and others, the dire consequences of giving confusing messages to a child. The adult in therapy is in a comparably vulnerable position. He needs to be able to trust in the coherence of the experience that the therapist brings to him. If the therapist, for example, denies that he has an emotion which the patient has sensed intuitively, the latter will become uncertain of the validity of his own perceptions with dangerous consequences to his psychic strength. Similarly, if the therapist, by omitting to respond, implies that his patient's moral outlook is of no concern to him yet clearly abhors his blatant racism, a comparable and harmful confusion can easily occur. This much seems obvious, but the subject of moral neutrality involves further questions. Our views on how we should be to one another in general will have a bearing on what kind of relationship we seek with our patients. Should they adapt to our way of working or try to change it? Do we believe in caution or spontaneity, in reticence or openness? How intimate do we try to become with our patients? What risks do we feel are justified—on both sides—in attempting to provoke intimacy? To what degree is our theory and method a rationalization of our own deeply held assumptions about what constitutes a good way to relate? Do we believe that people should readily turn to professional workers or should they seek them out only when the situation is desperate and all ordinary sources of help have failed? On many such issues even the therapist is groping in the dark and can only hope that his views are not hopelessly misguided—deeply held assumptions and prejudices about life. There is no higher authority to turn to in these matters. In the absence of such authority it would seem honest for the therapist to confront the fact of morality quite openly: to accept and admit that he does live by a moral sense and that he recognizes that any difference between the two people on moral questions has a bearing on the therapy. It then becomes possible for a discussion to occur in which both therapist and patient can consider their own and the other's beliefs on as equal a footing as is possible in the circumstances. As a consequence, the patient may be able to free himself from seeing the therapist as an authoritarian judge who will tell him how to live or an adversary with whom he may have to struggle in order to retain his integrity.

References

1. Ingleby, D. (1980). *Critical psychiatry: The politics of mental health*, p. 27 .Pantheon, New York.
2. Roazen, P. (1996). Erich Fromm's courage. In *A prophetic analyst* (ed. M. Cortina, M. Jacoby, and M. Fironson), p. 440. Aronson, Northvale.
3. Rieff, P. (1965). *The mind of the moralist*. Methuen, London.
4. Brunner, J. (1995). *Freud and the politics of psychoanalysis*. Blackwell, Oxford.
5. Jones, E. (1953–7). *The life and work of Sigmund Freud*, Vol. 2 p. 182. Basic Books, New York. (Quoted by Brunner, J., op. cit., p. 80.)
6. Money-Kyrle, R. E. (1995). Psychoanalysis and ethics. In *New directions in psychoanalysis*, (ed. M. Klein, P. Heimann, and R. E. Money-Kyrle) p. 421. Tavistock, London.
7. Hinshelwood, R. D. (1997). *Therapy or coercion: Does psychoanalysis differ from brainwashing?* Karnac, London.
8. Symington, N. (1994). *Emotion and spirit. Questioning the claims of psychoanalysis and religion*. Cassell, London.
9. Ibid., p. 130.
10. Symington, N. (1996). *The making of a psychotherapist*, p. xvi. Karnac, London.

11. Lomas, P. (1981). *The case for a personal psychotherapy.* Oxford University Press. (Republished as *The psychotherapy of everyday life.* Transaction, New Brunswick, NJ.)

12. Aron, L. (1996). *A meeting of minds: Mutuality in psychoanalysis.* Analytic Press, London.

13. Ferenczi, S. (1988). *The Clinical Diary of Sandor Ferenczi,* (ed. J. Dupont, trans. M. Balint, and N. Z. Jackson), p. 94. Harvard University Press, Cambridge, MA.

14. Holmes, J. and Lindley, R. (1989). *The values of psychoanalysis.* Oxford University Press. (1989)

4

Moral influence

The passions, lifestyles, and morals of human beings—especially of the people with whom we deal daily—continue to affect us at a deeper level. We revolt against those whom we hate while impressions left by those whom we love blend gently into our nature. We become accustomed to the voice, mien, glance and expression of the other in such a way that we unconsciously appropriate them and transmit them to others.

Johann Gottfried Herder

In the previous chapter I suggested that the contemporary psychotherapist evades the issue of his or her moral influence on the patient. This is not, I think, in doubt. The real difficulty comes when one tries to think about how best moral questions should be addressed and what justifications can be made for attempting to influence the other morally in an open way.

The dangers of making dogmatic moral assertions ('I think you should do *this* rather than *that*') are all too obvious. There are already too many people around who tell us how we should behave yet have little claim to wisdom in these matters. It is, however, another matter to attempt to elucidate moral issues: to tease out, in the manner of Socrates, the reasons for and consequences of certain actions. How useful to us are moral philosophers in such a quest? In writing this book I have turned to certain philosophical teachings in the hope of clarifying my thoughts and have found them of help. But the preoccupation with logic characteristic of philosophic thinking can sometimes lead us very far astray; logic is a fallible guide as to how to live.

The therapist is in a different situation from the philosopher. Her stance is more humble for she need make no claim to speak with authority on general issues. She is, however, in a very good position to elucidate issues that concern another person, and will, in time, become very practised at it. It is likely that, being thrust into the midst of moral dilemmas, day in and day out, she will become interested in generalities (and may be tempted to write about them) but her focus is the unique ('What would be best for *this* person at *this* time in *this* situation?'). Her position is also different from that of a judge in law who, although similarly practised in elucidating specific moral issues, is concerned with whether an action conforms to a particular, well-defined, code of practice, and who is confident of the correctness of this code. (She does, however, share one advantage with the judge; she is given permission to ask questions which, in most situations, would be thought impertinent.)

One kind of practitioner whose task, in some respects, is not unlike that of the therapist is the novelist. The great novelists, according to Martha Nussbaum, are concerned with quality rather than quantity, the particular rather than the general. With their gifts, dedication, and concentration they portray ordinary living with a precision that the rest of us cannot match.

The novelist's terms are even more variegated, more precise in their qualitative rightness, than are the sometimes blunt vague terms of daily life: they show us vividly what we can aspire to in refining our (already qualitative) understanding.[1]

Nussbaum maintains that the novel is deeply concerned with the presentation of choices between qualitatively different actions and, in order to do this adequately—to understand the pervasiveness of such conflicts in human efforts to live well—requires 'commitment over a relatively long time'.

The therapist is similarly required to show the life of a person in its complexity without relying on stereotypes for her perception, and like the novelist, need not claim to have privileged access to the truth or to lead a life that is superior to those for whom she works. But both professions require of their practitioners the possession of a certain degree of perceptiveness, imagination, patience, and a passionate interest in what they are doing.

The differences between the task of the therapist and that of the novelist are obvious. The psychotherapist is exploring an actual individual with whom she has a direct relationship and uses her imagination in a different way: the drama is enacted in immediate reality. Moral questions can only be explored to the extent that is relevant to the patient's good. Paths which might impersonally arouse her curiosity or may be intellectually satisfying cannot be pursued regardless of the reason why the two people are in the room in the first place. The novelist is free from these restrictions to the reaches of her imaginative power. Nevertheless, the therapist can learn from the novelist's art.

Nussbaum, whose guide in this matter is Aristotle, writes that:

The Aristotelian conception contains a view of learning well suited to support the claims of literature. For teaching and learning, here, do not simply involve the learning of rules and principles. A large part of learning takes place in the experience of the concrete. This experiential learning, in turn, requires the cultivation of perception and responsiveness: the ability to read a situation, singling out what is relevant for thought and action. This active task is not a technique; one learns it by guidance rather than by a formula. [Henry] James plausibly suggests that novels exemplify and offer such learning: exemplify it in the efforts of the characters and the author, engender it in the reader by setting up a similarly complex activity.

There is a further way in which novels answer to an Aristotelian view of practical learning. The Aristotelian view stresses that bonds of close friendship or love (such as those that connect members of a family, or close personal friends) are extremely important in the whole business of becoming a good perceiver. Trusting the guidance of a friend and allowing one's feelings to be engaged with that other person's life and choices, one learns to see aspects of the world that one had previously missed.[2]

An opposite question posed by Nussbaum is: 'Why can't we investigate whatever we want to investigate by living and reflecting on our lives?' Her answer is that, of course, we do so, but our lives are confined to our immediate experience whereas literature enables us to expand this; moreover, in the activity of literary imagining we are led to imagine and describe with greater precision, focusing our attention on each word, feeling each event more keenly—whereas much of actual life goes by without such heightened awareness, and is thus, in a certain sense, not fully or thoroughly lived.[3]

Although there is substance in Nussbaum's conception we should, I believe, view it with some circumspection. The term 'heightened awareness', for example, is certainly applicable to the practice of good psychotherapy but suggests a rather solemn and precious conversation rather than one that can be heated, harrowing, messy, or fun. If the therapist were to speak as Henry James writes we would be in a world remote from ordinary living. It would be a mistake to elevate either literature or psychotherapy to a higher realm than that of everyday life despite the fact that certain experiences can occur in these fields which are not readily available elsewhere.

What part, we may ask, does the patient play in the elucidation of moral dilemmas? Although, insofar as he resists insight he presents an obstacle to moral truth, he may also facilitate it. Not only may his genuine urge to be a better person provoke him to join with the therapist in an effort to tease out the truth, but the sheer intractability of his desperate attempt to preserve his stance in life may create crises which force the therapist to reconsider her own stance.

The psychotherapist's task in relation to moral dilemmas is not necessarily completed by elucidating them. May she not be justified, at times, in voicing her own opinion? And may her passion play a part in the encounter? Although doctors, engineers, plumbers, and lawyers do, unfortunately, give wrong advice, they can claim that, having studied the subject, they are in a better position than the rest of us to come up with a useful opinion. The psychotherapist, as I have suggested, is on much less secure ground. In view of this fact it would seem fitting that any advice she may give would be presented with a good measure of humility. To put it another way, if both people are faced with complexities beyond their full comprehension, the views of either of them are deserving of respect. This is in contrast to the situation in which an engineer comes to repair my television set. I would hope that he would treat me with respect as a human being and would listen carefully to my complaint but, unless I had engineering experience myself, he would not be very impressed if I suggested that the pink wires go one way and the blue ones another way. The patient, however, knows a lot about the 'wires' inside him and the world in which he operates and it would be presumptuous of the therapist to assume that she knows better. When the two discuss the patient's problem and disagree, the latter could be right even though he is a patient, even though he may have never heard of Freud, and even though he may be hospitalized and diagnosed as a 'paranoid schizophrenic'.

The attitude of humility that would seem appropriate for psychotherapy is, I believe, of a different quality from the philosophical dictum that all views on morality (on how we should live) are merely declarations of preference and have no bearing on things as they are. To hold such a view may sometimes make us aware of the limitations of mankind's understanding, but it is so unlike the way we actually behave in daily life that it hardly impinges upon us. Indeed, those who hold this view, far from showing humility, not infrequently are arrogant in their dismissal of the 'naïve' opinion of the man-in-the-street. Later, I shall discuss some of the arguments against moral relativism; at this point I simply note that, both in and out of the consulting room, people act as though they believe in objective good and bad.

Certain kinds of behaviour are so striking that most people have no difficulty in taking a moral position. There are, I imagine, few practitioners who would advocate savage mutilation of children as a sporting pastime or would rest content if their patients became serial killers. There are, however, cultural conventions and political or religious practices that are absolutely binding for some yet arbitrary or distasteful to others; and it is in these grey areas that therapist and patient will, from time to time, come into conflict. If the therapist wishes to influence the patient in certain ways what degree of force, if any, is justified? Is she justified in using powerful intellectual arguments to convince the patient of her own viewpoint? Can the discussion be on an equal basis, given the vulnerability of the patient's position and the practised strength of the therapist, who although unlikely to be more intelligent than the patient is in an accustomed role? Should she hide a passionately held viewpoint or would it be more useful, more honest, more human, to reveal her cards and say, 'I don't believe that is a good way of living'?

I have made a distinction between behaviour that is elemental in that it is likely to provoke universal approval or disapproval and, on the other hand, behaviour that is a matter of convention. But, although the distinction is often significant it is not always clear-cut. What is conventional is not necessarily trivial. Many of the attitudes to life which affect us most deeply and give us a sense of identity are embedded in our culture; we take them in during childhood as we take in a language—yet we do not necessarily have to reject them in order to find ourselves. For this reason the therapist who, following the ideas of Erikson, Laing, Winnicott, and others, seeks the 'true self', has to rely on her intuition in teasing out whether the voice rings true. How someone manages to evolve an authentic self—one that is neither a thoughtless acceptance of dogma nor a compulsive reaction against it—is a mystery, but it is a mystery similar to the existence of a faculty we call 'free will'. Nevertheless, an assessment of whether the patient's moral stance is a true expression of his being is central to any therapeutic undertaking. Although Freud conceived the matter in different terms this issue was the foundation stone of his work; put negatively, he devised a method of spotting the patient's inauthenticity. We are dealing here with a disposition, namely, integrity, which most people, I imagine, would regard as a virtue. Insofar as the therapist aims to cultivate this in her patient she is trying to influence him to be a good person. As with all questions of morality the situation is a complex one: much depends on how one defines integrity. We can all too easily remain so dedicated to maintaining a certain ideal of behaviour that we do so to the detriment of ourselves and to others. A virtue can be debased if it is pursued at the expense of the whole.

Mankind has a tendency towards specialization, and consequently a retreat from wholeness. No body of men have a greater passion for pursuing distinctions than Western philosophers. Descartes, with a force comparable to that of splitting the atom, separated thought from action, soul from body, and self from other. Although this fragmentation still has a powerful hold over us, many voices have now been raised in protest. The list includes those of Polyani, MacMurray, the existentialists and, more recently, Bohm, MacIntyre, and Midgeley. I will return to this matter in Chapter 10. At this point I want to consider the fragmentation of our moral sense.

John MacMurray starts from the existentialist view that the philosophical problem of the present century is the crisis of the personal, and maintains that it can only be usefully approached by an attempt 'to discover or to construct the intellectual form of the personal'.[4] We live, he believes, in an age of abrogation of personal responsibility involving 'the subordination of the personal aspect of human life to its functional aspect'. The self is not, in MacMurray's view, a knower or a thinker, but a doer, an 'agent':

> Action, then is a full concrete activity of the self in which all our capacities are employed; while thought is constituted by the exclusion of some of our powers and a withdrawal into an activity which is less concrete and less complete.[5]

Because we are agents our prime purpose is how best to *act*. We cannot be indifferent to the truth *but* 'the distinction between "true" and "false" is secondary'.

Alasdair MacIntyre, who is a much more influential writer than MacMurray, comes to not dissimilar conclusions about the primacy of the moral world. He approaches the matter by the historical route, and sets out to save us 'from the new dark ages which are already upon us and to reinstate the concept of virtue which was at the centre of Aristotelian ethics'.[6] MacIntyre maintains that debate on moral issues is conducted in a style that renders it fruitless, for the 'rival premises are such that we possess no rational way of weighing the claims of one as against the other'.[7] The consequence is either interminable argument or retreat into an apathetic acceptance of the belief that there is no valid basis for solid evaluation and that we should therefore rely on non-moral ways of settling problems. Either approach is ineffective in dealing with the world. The predominant contemporary moral philosophy makes a sharp distinction between ends and means, apportioning good only to ends (insofar as it is accepted that there is such a thing as good) and relegating means to a non-moral, technical area of existence. MacIntyre will have no such distinction. We best understand goodness, he believes, by seeing

it in action and we best articulate its nature not by crude rules
and procedures, but by stories, for stories are concrete and try
to do justice to the uniqueness of the person and his circumstances.

If my understanding of MacIntyre is correct, then his diagnosis aptly applies to the current plight of psychotherapy; or,
to put it another way, contemporary psychotherapy is a particular example and endorsement of MacIntyre's general
hypothesis. It is perhaps significant that student therapists are
warned by their teachers to avoid getting into an intellectual
argument with patients, for to do so lends support to their
'intellectual defence'. It could be the case that the intellectual
defence and the contemporary poverty of intellectual debate
about moral issues are two sides of the same coin.

MacIntyre's conception of morality lends support to the idea
that the therapist is mistaken in thinking that procedures in
themselves can lead someone towards a better life. Because
each situation is unique, the therapist has no special authority
to define what should be done and, if she wishes to influence
the patient for good she can only rely on her own moral sense,
where relevant, and convey this sense to the patient.

I will end this chapter with a few brief descriptions of conversations in therapy with the aim of illustrating some of the
ways in which a therapist may attempt to influence the client
to be a better person. These bits of dialogue do not prove anything or convey a procedure that should be followed. But perhaps, like the stories to which MacIntyre refers, they may
express something that I cannot manage discursively.

Paul told me of a recent occasion when he had behaved
'without any dignity'. He was clearly distressed and ashamed
of himself. I listened to the details and agreed that he had, indeed, behaved without dignity.

I would find it hard to justify this response in terms of accepted analytic theory, but it had the merit of validating his
own moral perception (which I believed to be justified) and
helping him to face it. It may be that an interpretation or exploration ('Why do you think that you acted in this way?')
would have achieved the same result by conveying the implication that his behaviour was poor and required understanding and 'treatment'. But we cannot be sure of this. Moreover,
the quick move to explanation may have enabled him to avoid

the experience of shame by focusing on an intellectual search. Whatever the pros and cons of my response it is clearly one that is quite openly in the realm of morality: I agreed that his behaviour was to be deplored and in so doing I confessed my own moral view on the matter of dignity.

Towards the end of the session we discussed his past relationship with his parents and the bearing of this on what he now called his lack of 'manliness'. The change from 'dignity' to 'manliness' again introduced the question of moral values, for it seemed necessary to attempt to tease out the relationship between the two terms. At one point, when he was expressing helplessness and castigating himself in a useless way I sensed that our discussion was getting nowhere. I then brought up the matter of my own lack of influence on him. Why had I not been, as yet, able to help him become more manly? I suggested that there was more to it than a failure on my part to engender a fruitful account of his life-experience, and that it had something to do with our relationship—a distorted perception on his part or some unsatisfactory attitude on mine. At one point I said that I liked and respected him and added, with what I think was probably a wry grin, 'despite the failings we've just been talking about'.

The implication (at least for me) of this discussion is that it could be expected that someone who turns to another in a relationship of mutual respect may well be influenced by the latter's moral stance and behaviour. Although I made my comment in the context of probing into how we thought we behaved towards each other, I think I had another motive. I felt that I could now, later in the session, safely give him some reassurance to counteract a sense of shame which had been experienced quite deeply.

Another patient, Richard, spoke of his reluctance to confront his sister who was making a lot of difficult demands on him. 'She *is* difficult', he said, 'but I know that I never expect any results from confronting anyone. Either I feel they won't listen to me or, if I really confront them, they will be wounded'. After some discussion about this I said:

> 'I think that you don't confront me and you seduce me into not confronting you. We get on very well and much of it is fun, but it's all too comfortable. Whatever I say doesn't really shake you and you don't try to shake me.'

'Yes. When you criticize me I think, "Yes, he's right. I *am* like
   that", but it doesn't hurt me as much as when someone criticizes my writing.'
'That implies that it's your writing that is valuable, not you.'
'I suppose it does. As long as I can entertain people and write
   well I feel I'm OK. It's never occurred to me to think otherwise.'

In this conversation I question his value system, hoping that
he will come to base his self-respect on new criteria—those in
which I myself believe. The matter could, of course, be put in
psychoanalytic terms, omitting any reference to value, for example, that Richard has effected a displacement from sense of
self as a whole to an aspect of self; or, that there is an idealization, for whatever reason, of the qualities of literary gifts and
the capacity to be amusing. To put it this way implies a value
judgement but does not express it openly—indeed, the therapist following psychoanalytic tradition would be likely to deny
having expressed a value judgement. Yet in making the point
to Richard I called attention to values which are basic to my
sense of life, have a long philosophical and religious tradition
behind them, and which I would have been quite prepared to
discuss with Richard had he questioned them.

   Later in the session, we turn to his perennial expectation of
disappointment. 'I never seem to learn,' he said. 'Even if things
do turn out well it doesn't make any difference next time.' I
suggested that any favourable outcome made no difference
because he felt so bitter about life, and had felt this way for so
long, that he was not prepared to take the risk of disappointment.

'But I don't know *how* to do it,' he said.
'I don't think it's a question of how, I think it's a question of your
   preparedness to give it a go, to take the risk.'

Once again, I am not claiming that my comment was particularly apt, but I believe it is justifiable, at some point, to suggest
that we are dealing with a moral question ('Have I the bottle?
Do I dare? Should I forgive?'), and to encourage him to believe
that a better way of living is open to him.

   Frieda was feeling angry because of a great disappointment;
she and a friend had been planning a project but, then, quite
suddenly, the friend pulled out.

'I hope she suffers for it: I really hope she suffers and then is
sorry.' Frieda said. 'It's normal to feel like that isn't it? Isn't that
human nature?'

'Yes, I think so. But it's a matter of degree. Do you think it's her
fault? Don't you think she too might be disappointed?'

'No, I understand why she pulled out. I don't really think she's
behaved badly.'

'But your feelings imply this. There's no compassion alongside
the anger.'

We talked a bit about her tendency to vengefulness. I suggested that she felt she had a divine right to have things her
way. I pointed out how she had tended, at times, to be furious
with me if there was an interruption, or if I seemed to be not
attending a hundred per cent.

'Actually,' she said, 'I was rather proud of getting angry with
someone I was a bit frightened of. Isn't that what's meant to be
therapeutic? I used to be so compliant when I was younger.'

'I take your point. I think that's fine. But it doesn't mean that
when you express anger in therapy it's necessarily creative—
that we put out the flags and rejoice and say therapy is working. It could be an aspect of spoiltness.'

'Yes. I agree. It may be an excuse, but often being suppressed so
much of my life I feel now, here's a chance, take it; and I've a
lot to make up for. I want to grab everything. I'm greedy for
everything.'

'I don't think you're simply excusing yourself. I think that's quite
an admission. It certainly doesn't put you morally in the clear.'

'No, it doesn't. It makes me feel not a nice person. You've been
nudging at this for ages, but I took no notice. But when I look
at what I've done I feel awful.'

As she left, Frieda picked up my newspaper, which was on a
chair. 'Now, I'm feeling nosy,' she said. 'I'm looking at this picture of a glamorous woman. Who is she?'

'I've no idea.'

'You see. I want everything. I want to be glamorous, like her.'

On reading this interchange again I am struck by Frieda's
good-natured and undefensive acceptance of my criticism. If
people were always like that the therapist's task would be
much easier. What is difficult is to be able to give the reasons
why I think the conversation was creative rather than barren;
to do so convincingly would require a detailed description of
the therapy over a number of years, a process which had re-

sulted in a slow increase of respect, liking, and trust in each other. Because of this change, criticisms could be made, on either side, without either of us feeling too hurt by them.

Finally, I will relate an interchange described to me by a colleague to whom I was confessing my hesitation in bringing in the concept of morality when talking about psychotherapy. She immediately recounted the following episode:

A man who had herpes on his penis told me that he had unprotected sex with a young woman, concealing his affliction from her. Although quite aware of the danger to her he was unrepentant. 'I couldn't resist a good fuck!', he said.

I am embarrassed to say that I lost my temper. Perhaps I identified with the woman because I am the same sex. But the sheer callousness, selfishness, and complacency were more than I could bear. I told him exactly what I thought of him and I was quite emotionally charged. I talked about how, in my view, people should behave to each other.

At the end of the session the man was crying helplessly, aghast that he could have done such a thing. And he cried, off and on, for a week. "No one", he said, "has ever spoken to me like that before." But the session changed him and his attitude to others, and this has remained so. I think that one thing that affected him was that he realized I was interested in him. As a child he felt no one was really interested.

The therapist's response was spontaneous and intuitive; it came from the heart. There was no question of technique. It was honest and courageous and made by someone whose moral sense on this issue was sound, and I would guess that these qualities in the response made their mark.

References

1. Nussbaum, M. (1990). *Love's knowledge: Essays on philosophy and literature*. Oxford University Press.
2. Ibid., p. 44.
3. Ibid., p. 47.
4. MacMurray, J. (1957). *The self as agent*, p. 29. Faber, London.
5. Ibid., p. 89.
6. MacIntyre, A. (1985). *After virtue: A study in moral theory*, p. 263. Duckworth, London.
7. Ibid., p. 8.

5

The poverty of technique

But, after all, for thousands and thousands of years people have been led to believe that anything and everything can be obtained if only one had the right techniques and methods. What is needed is to be aware of the care with which the mind slips comfortably back into this age-old pattern.

David Bohm

The justification for bureaucratic procedures resides not in any argument in support of intrinsic values but in their capacity to effect the result that is desired. The question as to whether the desire is a good one is bypassed. In discussing these issues, MacIntyre[1] compares the manager with the therapist who also:

treats ends as given, as outside his scope; his concern also is with technique, with effectiveness in transforming neurotic symptoms into directed energy, maladjusted individuals well-adjusted ones. Neither manager nor therapist, in their roles as manager and therapist, are able to engage in moral debate. They are seen by themselves, and by those who see them with the same eyes as their own, as un-contested figures, who purport to restrict themselves to the realms in which rational agreement is possible—that is, of course, from their point of view to the realm of fact, the realm of means, the realm of measurable effectiveness.[2]

If MacIntyre's diagnosis is right—and, despite much criticism of the detail, his main thesis has survived well—it presents a challenge to our profession.[3]

One of the problems that confronts the psychotherapist is the basis on which he can justify his practice. As a bureaucrat, he will try to support it by results that can be succinctly formulated. This is an endeavour that can seem possible for those approaches which depend on technical measures with well-defined and limited aims (e.g. cognitive therapy). For those of us who are less sure of our precise aims but seek, yet question, the meaning of what might be a richer life for our patients, the public justification for what we do is a formidable task. Freud's position is confused: he was able to find meaning where others had seen only mechanism, but he never freed himself from the mechanistic approach of his neurological background. His theory could not encompass the fact that what occurs in the consulting room is, like all human relationships, unpredictable.

The practice of a technique results in simplification. There are certain lines of action considered desirable or necessary and others which are to be avoided. For example, I once reported as part of a conversation with a patient that I did not think her a 'horrible' person, as she maintained, adding: 'I think I know how you feel. Sometimes at 3 a.m. I become aware of what a narcissistic, ambitious, egotistical person I am, and I despair of myself. But I know it's not all of me. You're forgetting the loving part of yourself . . .' A reviewer (who was a psychoanalyst) made the comment that I was guilty of faulty technique and went on to say that she regarded such a response as 'never being suitable for any patient, under any circumstances'. I could, I hope, accept that my words may have been unwise, inappropriate, clumsy, unhelpful, or plain stupid—that they failed to match up to this particular occasion. But to say this is quite different from judging it as being wrong because it does not match up to a particular theory.

Although we may not wish to endorse a rule of restraint in therapy there is clearly some merit in recommending that we do not indulge thoughtlessly in self-revelations, thereby failing to give due attention to the other person. If, however, the therapist possesses any degree of humility he is not likely to do this. Lack of humility cannot be adequately replaced by what one might call a 'technique of healing by self-revelation'—a method that could be learnt from a book. There is no technique for behaving well towards another person.

Therapeutic technique has something in common with a code of manners. The dividing line between an act of courtesy performed out of generosity or one undertaken because it is regarded as acceptable behaviour is often difficult to identify. One would not nowadays readily say: 'A number of people were killed but they were only niggers'. But the reluctance to do so may come either from an avoidance of being thought politically incorrect or from a deep-seated respect for the value of human beings irrespective of colour, sex, or social class. Good manners, if not carried to excess, can be a useful guideline in managing certain social situations but lack the depth and flexibility that comes from a simple respect for others. And psychotherapeutic technique may serve a comparable purpose in therapy, helping the therapist, particularly in the early stages of his or her career, to get by. But it is not the stuff of which good therapy is made.

Technique is, in a sense, too easy. It tempts us along known paths along which we can travel with confidence but turns our eyes away from the surrounding countryside. To give an example, a woman was talking about the unsatisfactoriness of those around her; they were, in her view, insensitive and lacking in understanding. In looking for a response there were two obvious suggestions that I might make: to put it in psychoanalytic terms, she was projecting her badness on to others and/or she was unconsciously deflecting transferential feelings towards me. To follow either or both these paths may have been rewarding and I could have immediately made interpretations to this effect.

But there are other paths, of a more ordinary nature, that could be followed. I have no idea whether, in choosing a different path, I was wise or not. In fact, we discussed, in detail, the nature of her complaints and tried to assess their validity. This involved us in a wide-ranging conversation including, for example, the relationships of men and women, the bringing up of children, teaching, politics, class differences, cliques, her style of communicating, how she and I communicated and so on. The fact that I know, having learnt it from Freud, that people can project and transfer experiences from the past on to present day relationships ensured that at some point, if not in this session, I would think of these possibilities. This knowledge is one item among everything I have learnt about life and is not essentially different from the rest of what I know. I am not assuming that those who claim to work by means of psychoanalytic technique would not bring all their experience of living and their sensitivity to the manner and timing of interpretations to the encounter, but, insofar as they keep theory and technique in their minds they would be likely to pursue a style suited to the implementation of orthodox interpretations, inevitably narrowing the range of their feedback to the patient. I suspect that there are many psychoanalysts who are sparing in their use of interpretations and who may have responded to my patient in a way not unlike mine; but if this is the case they are not practising a technique.

Whether a comment in psychotherapy is likely to be considered to be a technical move or a moral statement is often a matter of the words used. The essential message may be the same, although the articulation will convey different implications in each case. I will give an example.

I commented to a woman that in talking about her life she seemed stuck in a groove:

'How do I get out of it?'
'I think we only advance if we take risks.'
'What risks?'
'Well, what are you most afraid of happening'
'Finding out that I'm an awful person.'
'Perhaps you are an awful person. What's the big deal? Not many of us are angels.'

I could have said: 'Yes, I think you are afraid of the destructiveness in you.' Although hardly an interpretation this confirmation of the source of her anxiety would have conformed to psychoanalytic theory and terminology and therefore could be considered a technical mode of presentation. In using the words I've reported I overtly placed the discussion in the moral realm. As she left, the patient said, 'I like it when you talk seriously'. I did not ask her what she meant. My guess is that she was referring to my openness about morality.

It is the view of John Heaton that it would be better to conceive psychotherapy as a practice rather than a technique. Technique is inadequate, he believes, because we thereby:

make representations of the end we desire and then devise the most efficient means to attain it. We define the end within a system of concepts and then devise the means to reach that end, the whole process remaining by necessity within the system of concepts.

Medical practice is technical in this way. If we become ill we have a picture of what health is, which is usually the state we were in before we became ill. The doctor then devises means to restore us to that state as quickly and comfortably as possible.[4]

Heaton maintains that there is a long tradition in philosophy and medicine which argues that practice is more fundamental than theory or knowledge. Practice is concerned with efficacy rather than rationality:

In practice, the "feel for the game" is all important; the way things unfold in time, rhythm, tempo and directionality is constitutive of meaning . . . One may have a marvellous sense of timing in tennis but not in politics or even golf. Theory has a time but it is not that of practice. The theoretician knows what has happened, he sees all, so he can totalize. The player who is involved adjusts not to what he sees but to what he foresees; he anticipates. He decides in response to the overall, instantaneous assessment of the situation; "on the spot", "in the twinkling of an eye", "in the heat of the moment". These are terms which are more expressive and accurate than hosts of theoretical ones. It is the ability to make these finely honed responses with genuineness that is at the heart of psychotherapy.[5]

The influence of the Enlightenment has led to a rejection of traditional thinking and its replacement by fields of knowledge in which practice became subordinate to theory and knowledge. This new outlook enabled Freud to claim to have founded a rational and scientific discipline, discarding the traditional notions of trust and faith. Heaton believes that psychoanalysts, as Enlightenment thinkers, 'assumed psychoanalysis was superior to their own parental power'. He contrasts this attitude to that of Galen, who noted that the upbringing of infants and children affects later life and attempted to heal through discourse, including attention to dreams. Galen thought that it was the insight and attentiveness of the therapist that was important and recommended that he use his passions to combat disorder:

Psychotherapy has a long tradition and its origins, like those of any deep tradition, are lost in the mists of time. For human beings have a natural desire to tend and help those who are in pain and distress and this desire is the source from which flows the practice of medicine and psychotherapy.[6]

In her study of Hellenic philosophy[7] Martha Nussbaum shows that the thinkers regarded their work as a practice, a moral pursuit, and therapy, and calls attention to their emphasis of the uniqueness of the individual and the positive role of passion in true vision. She reminds us of the view of Epicurus:

Empty is that philosopher's pursuit by which no human suffering is therapeutically treated. For just as there is no use in a medical art that does not cast out the sicknesses of bodies, so too there is no use in philosophy, if it does not throw out suffering from the soul.[8]

Nussbaum asserts that:

Asking how to live is never, in Greek tradition, a merely academic exercise, nor philosophy a merely academic subject. It is prompted by real human perplexities, and it must address these in the end. But the Hellenistic schools move well beyond Aristotle, and even beyond Socrates and Plato, in their fine-tuned attention to the interlocutor's concrete needs and motives for philosophizing. They design their procedures so as to engage those deepest motivations and speak to those needs. The different schools do this in different ways, with rather different conceptions of the diseases that lead the pupil to seek the philosophical doctor. Yet from all of these attempts contemporary moral philosophy has much to learn, if it wishes to move beyond the academy to take its place in the daily lives of human beings.[9]

Although technique is an inadequate and inappropriate way of conceiving psychotherapy it can have its uses under certain conditions (e.g. short-term work or moments of crisis). In most walks of life we find it helpful to have a few strategies or ploys up our sleeve which enable us to get by when we are at a loss. In games, particularly chess, one may lull the opponent into making a rash move, and, in football, we may develop a technique for appearing to make a pass without carrying it out. Such manoeuvres constitute deception and trickery, but this does not mean that they are necessarily immoral; if they were, our capacity to have fun and to joke would be sadly impoverished. It would therefore be illogical to maintain that they cannot have a useful place in psychotherapy, provided that they are not considered to be the essence of the procedure: in other words, the therapist may joke or play tricks on his patient in a way that does not invalidate trust and openness. But what of those therapies which place such gambits at the centre of the work?

Let us take, for example, the technique of the 'paradoxical injunction', a manoeuvre developed by family systems therapy, by means of which an instruction places a family or an individual in an ambiguous position, thereby blocking any obvious, logical, or reasonable response. This tactic was developed from the work of Gregory Bateson, whose influential theory of the 'double bind' showed the way in which a child can become confused to the point of extreme mental disturbance by being given contradictory messages. Hoffman[10] gives an example of a parent saying to an adolescent: 'I want you to be independent. But I want you to want that independently of my wanting that'.

Depending on the circumstances, a paradoxical injunction may lead either to pathology or emancipation. The child trapped in a family can find no escape; but in other situations a 'creative leap' can be possible. Hoffman likens this therapeutic endeavour to that of the Zen master who holds a stick in front of a student and says: 'Here is a stick. If you say it is real I will hit you with it. If you say it is not real I will hit you with it. If you say nothing I will hit you with it'. A creative move by the student might be to take the stick away.[11]

This kind of policy has a risk comparable to that of the patient in psychoanalysis who, under the influence of transference, feels herself to be in the anguished situation of a childhood dilemma she could not solve; one hopes for a better outcome this time, but this is not guaranteed. From the point of view of this discussion, the question is whether the problem to be addressed is so intransigent that the therapist is justified in indulging in deception. As a kind of shock treatment, a manoeuvre that, in family therapy, is often referred to as 'crisis intervention', a good case can be made for it. But it is less easy to justify in long-term therapy, which depends so much on the gradual growth of mutual trust, honesty, and openness.

Although the psychotherapy of which I write has as its most immediate source of inspiration the work of Freud, it also has affinities with all those efforts, throughout history, through which someone attempts to understand, support, encourage, and console a person in distress. A better word for what I have in mind is 'counselling'. It has a simple, ordinary, human, existential quality. It is not itself a technique, although it is usually thought to be. Those therapies which overtly place techniques at the centre of the enterprise, for example, behaviour therapy and cognitive therapy—stand in contrast to counselling as I am using the word. Not only do they have a different approach but their aim is usually a different one. They can achieve results that cannot readily be achieved by the counsellor; and vice versa. And just as the counsellor will sometimes use ploys, so will the 'technical' therapist rely on counselling, a fact which is beginning to be recognized.

Theories and techniques can give immense impetus to a quest to understand the nature of relationships. What Bateson's theory of the double-bind accomplished, I believe, was a neat, though inadequate, formula which had the enormous merit of drawing our attention to the ways in which people confuse each in the service of domination and self-preservation. But much of this confusion can now be better described in the subtleties of ordinary language. Many family therapists are now recognizing the limitations of technique and developing an approach which is more obviously based on attitudes that are part of everyday living.[12,13] My own experience of gifted family therapists leaves me with the impression that they rely on a substantial amount of common sense and ordinary wisdom. I will, in contrast, give an example of an intervention by a therapist which would, I believe, have been better conceived and undertaken in a less technical way.

A man with a stammer who took a job as a salesman was treated by 'strategic therapy':

His understandable belief that his speech problem would interfere with his ability to become a good salesman was challenged by the idea that, far from being a liability, his defect would be an asset. People always pay more attention to someone who has trouble talking, in contrast to the way they often turn off in response to a fast-talking huckster. Therefore this man was encouraged to increase his stammering as a way of becoming a better salesman. This is an example of the use of positive reframing in connection with prescribing the symptom. Clearly, in their clinical work the strategic therapists use a variety of therapeutic double binds and a variety of benevolent rationales for making them seem palatable.[14]

It would seem quite reasonable, in the course of ordinary conversation or therapy, to suggest to the man: 'Have you ever thought that your stammer may not, in some circumstances, be the disadvantage you believe it to be?' To present this idea as a special technique, however, is to give it an unwarranted authority. The term 'technique' would only be justified if limited to a method for cultivating his stammer. The man, we are given to understand, is prescribed a course of action rather as a physician might prescribe a drug. It has been decided, apparently, that the purpose of the therapy is to enable him to do this particular job more effectively and with more confidence. It may succeed, and could, in this particular case, be the best thing that could have happened to him at that moment. But we may have misgivings about the effect of deliberately increasing his stammer and thereby generating a dysfunctional action in the rest of his life.

If psychotherapy is not a technique a question arises as to whether the attempt to define and label it is a worthwhile pursuit. Those who practise it need to define their occupation to others for pragmatic purposes, but this may not amount to much more than the sort of answer one sometimes has to write on an official form which requests to know one's work, and the nearest answer is 'housewife', or 'househusband', or 'parent', or 'jack-of-all-trades'.

Recently, a colleague was talking about how he experienced his work. At one point he said: 'In my room I can make mistakes and it's acceptable; but outside, in the public world, I can't'. I wondered what light this threw on the nature of therapy. It is private. We are accountable to our patients and, for the most part, only to them. If we make mistakes, it is they who must forgive us or not; only they can really judge. The situation is similar to that between husband and wife, or between lovers: it is primarily their own affair, unless manifestly illegal behaviour or physical cruelty occurs. In short, it is personal. And because it is personal the moral qualities that contribute to a good relationship in ordinary life are also paramount in therapy. An example of the failure to give priority to moral considerations was given to me by a friend who told me that her therapist, in the interests of scrupulously following a technique, had held back important information thus risking serious, possibly fatal, harm to a third person.

In her book on Adolf Eichmann, Hannah Arendt[15] argues that his acts of atrocity were best seen as an example of the limitations of a bureaucratic attitude. The word 'banality', which appears in her subtitle, was, as Horowitz shows[16] the 'most appropriate single-word description of Adolf Eichmann'; and it was this word, perhaps more than anything that caused Arendt to offend so many of her readers, for at first sight the word appears to excuse Eichmann. I do not think it does so. Rather, it is a terrifying indictment of the evil that can result when the banality of bureaucracy (method, technique, operationalism) is separated from ordinary morality or given preference over it. If the consequences of idealizing technique in human situations can lead to such evil, we should perhaps pause before following it as freely as we do and wonder whether, even in circumstances such as that of psychotherapy, which are as far removed from that of Eichmann as can be imagined, it may be more disadvantageous than we realize. To speak of the two situations in the same breath may itself cause offence, but the most disparate of phenomena can have certain factors in common.

The limitation of technique is at no time more apparent than when the therapist is faced with naked grief, when someone is crying helplessly in the grip of an experience that is too painful for words, when the therapist can say nothing that would not seem presumptuous or trivial. Perhaps he might put an arm round the person; even that may seem not much of a thing to do. It could, however, be of some use if the despairing person feels to be in the presence of someone to whom, at that moment, any idea of a technical response would seem utterly foreign to the occasion. There seems no easy way of conveying such an occurrence in terms of what is usually meant by the term 'psychotherapy'.

The danger of saying or doing anything that might be taken as an underestimation of the intensity of grief is wonderfully portrayed in Robert Frost's poem *Home Burial*. The burial is that of a couple's child. The woman is grieving. We do not know how much later the scene takes place. The man, a farmer, is trying to console her; but whatever he says increases her alienation. She recalls the time when he dug the grave:

> I can repeat the very words you were saying,
> "Those foggy mornings and one rainy day
> Will rot the best birch fence a man can build."
> Think of it, talk like that at such a time!

What had how long it takes a birch to rot
To do with what was in the darkened parlour?
You couldn't care! The nearest friends can go
With anyone to death, comes so far short
They might as well not try to go at all.

Frost does not convey that the man's sensitivity or his experience of grief is necessarily of a trivial order; rather, the recognition that when someone is nakedly aware of the immeasurability of their grief, any attempt to lessen it, place it, normalize it (let alone interpret it) is likely to be felt as diminishing.

The tyranny of convention is the crushing force that lies behind inappropriate technique in psychotherapy. Under the sway of a belief in technique we tend to follow what is considered proper and respectable, what we can report to our colleagues or put into print without seeming naïve or irresponsibly reckless. Even more formidable, I think, is the dread of appearing to be sententious, sentimental, or pretentious if we try to describe our experience in terms other than that of technique. How can one convey the deep feeling that can be aroused when we manage to reach another's heart? We are not poets; we lack their gift, and we do not have their licence.

References

1. MacIntyre, A. (1985). *After virtue: A study in moral theory*. Duckworth, London.
2. Ibid., p. 30.
3. Horton, J. and Medus, S. (ed.) (1996). *After MacIntyre*. Polity Press, Oxford.
4. Heaton, J. M. (1993). The sceptical tradition in psychotherapy. In *From the words of my mouth: Tradition in psychotherapy*, (ed. L. Spurling), p. 114. Routledge, London.
5. Ibid., p. 121.
6. Ibid., p. 106.
7. Nussbaum, M. (1994). *The therapy of desire: Theory and practice in Hellenistic ethics*. Princetown University Press, Princeton, NJ.
8. Usener, H. (ed.) (1887). *Epicurea*, p. 221. Leipzig. (Quoted by Nussbaum, M., op. cit., p. 102.)
9. Nussbaum, M. op. cit., p. 486.

10. Hoffman, L. (1998). *Foundations of family therapy: A conceptual framework for systems change*, p. 168. Basic Books, New York.
11. Ibid., p. 168.
12. Ibid., p. 277.
13. Cecchin, G., Lane, G., and Ray. W. A. (1992). *Irreverence: A strategy for therapists' survival*. Karnac, London.
14. Asan, E. (1999). The limits of technique in family therapy. In *Committed uncertainty: Essays in honour of Peter Lomas*. (ed. L. King), pp. 120–36. Whurr, London.
15. Arendt, H. (1997). *Eichmann in Jerusalem: A report on the banality of evil*. Penguin, New York.
16. Horowitz, I. L. (1997). *Hannah Arendt: Juridical critic of totalitarianism*, Vol. 39, No. 4. Modern Age Intercollegiate Studies Institute, New Brunswick.

6

Spontaneity

Forced self-observations may become a severe handicap to the creativity of the artist. An attempt to produce on a conscious level what must grow in unconscious depths, the attempt to manipulate the primal creative process by reflecting on it, is doomed to failure.

Viktor Frankl

The further I continued in writing this book the more my heart sank. How can one possibly give a description of psychotherapy which bears sufficient resemblance to the actual article to make the account useful? When I think of some of the most fruitful occurrences in therapy I cannot relate them. This is not because I am ashamed of them. It is because they seem to have no more relevance to a professional undertaking based on a describable method than an account of a slice of life that might appear in a novel. They lack specificity; they do not form part of a planned approach; I do not know how to justify them as a therapeutic endeavour any more than conversations with friends which have been rewarding but from which no formula can be extracted for having rewarding conversations with friends. I refer to times when there is no conscious attempt to promote insight or strength in the other or to create a medium in which something therapeutic can occur. If these occasions were incidental to the undertaking then we do not have a serious conceptual problem. One would still be able to say that theory is the centrepiece of psychotherapy, whatever else may occur which contributes towards a desirable out-come. But this is not the case if significant benefit results from behaviour that is not designed to deliberately bring about a favourable change.

I write of my own experience and the convictions that have emerged from it; as the views of one particular therapist they carry little authority. I can find some support for them, how-ever, in the belief that they are based on the kind of relation-ship which might be expected to be creative. A rough account would be something as follows. (The attitude I shall describe would need to be present in both people for a good relation-ship to occur; it is difficult to achieve if one of the two is very inhibited, as, indeed, a seriously disturbed patient may well be. For the present, I shall confine myself to the attitude of the therapist.) To be of most help it would seem that, ideally, the therapist is flexible and balanced, enables us to feel we are in the presence of someone who is listening without prejudice, is free from an attempt to fit us into a formula, and who would not condemn us or convey a sense of superiority; there would be an atmosphere in which risks can be taken, fun can be had, closeness is possible, and the relationship feels alive. Some aspects of this approach would I think meet the criteria of what is often called the 'analytic attitude'; some would not. I can find no adequate word to describe this approach. Certain words—personal, ordinary, intuitive—go some way to indicat-ing the quality I have in mind. Another possibility is 'spon-taneous'.

The *Oxford English Dictionary* defines spontaneity as 'volun-tary', 'unconstrained', 'of one's own accord, freely, willingly'. But it also includes a definition with a markedly different em-phasis: 'without deep thought or meditation'. This ambiguity of meaning can very easily lead to a confusion about the word. It is surely admirable if one's actions are a genuine expression of oneself rather than a pretence. Spontaneity is that which comes out of a person without defensiveness, manipulation or calculation; it is being generous with the self. It is what Christ presumably had in mind when he spoke of giving without counting the cost and when he said: 'Consider the lilies of the field, how they grow' or: 'Whoever tries to save his life shall lose it'. It is the opposite of what psychoanalysts refer to as the 'anal character'. It implies a healthy self-confidence rather

than the self-preservative 'security operations' described by
Harry Stack Sullivan. It would seem, therefore, that to be
spontaneous is a good way of living. This is quite in contrast to
the usage of the word in order to describe egotistical, unthink-
ing, shallow, and precipitate behaviour. One factor which may
easily lead the therapist to be suspicious of spontaneity is the
belief, to which Freud subscribed, that the 'instinctive' behaviour of the child—and of the child in each of us—is narcissistic
and immoral and needs to be sharply brought into line. In contrast to Freud, Winnicott writes about the child's spontaneous
play with striking approval; it is, for him, the vital core of
being, to be encouraged and fostered. Winnicott, however,
had such loyalty to Freud and Klein that he never recognized
(or admitted) his radical departure from their beliefs. It is possibly for this reason that, despite his approval of spontaneity,
he was very reluctant to advocate it in therapy, except occasionally with very sick patients and in the hands of a very experienced therapist.

As an example of concentrated spontaneity I think of my
five-year-old granddaughter sitting, riveted, watching *Jungle
Book* on television. One could not easily see a more vibrant,
alive, unfettered human being. She was certainly listening
carefully, a fact which suggests that spontaneity may be far
from thoughtless or unreflective. When uninhibited our
minds can think very quickly: we call this faculty 'intuition';
many elements, conscious and unconscious, can be processed
in a flash. (Certainly, long deliberation about a problem can
bring immense benefits, but a constant attitude of careful con-
templation in the consulting room is not necessarily to the patient's advantage. Indeed, too much cautious consideration
may stem the flow of things.) A spontaneous, simple interest
in the world—that which a healthy child possesses—is not
necessarily narcissistic: it is concerned with other people.
Indeed, it is when we lose this simplicity, when we become
preoccupied with what others think of us, that we become
self-absorbed and narcissistic.

One can (readily) be spontaneously bad. The 'object–
relations' school of thought has not, I believe, come up with a
clear statement of an issue which has divided Western philosophy for many a year and which hinges on one's valuation
of emotion. Is the emotion which reveals itself in spontaneity

simply a healthy manifestation of vitality which is a potential for either good or bad? Or is it by definition bad and in need of restraint by another force, namely, reason? There is much to commend the former (non-Cartesian) concept. Cavell maintains that:

Experience is a co-operative exercise of spontaneity, drawing on our conceptual capacities and receptivity to the larger reality of which we are a part. We can abandon the view that spontaneity operates on some pre-conceptual "given", while keeping in mind that experience is an interplay between the world's acting on us in causal ways and our acting on the world.[1]

The extreme reluctance of psychotherapists to give due acknowledgement to the positive value of being spontaneous in sessions is, I believe, based on a philosophical error. Spontaneity may, like all action, be wise or foolish, but it is not necessarily thoughtless. Although it is extraordinarily difficult to formulate the nature of spontaneity one can perhaps say something about the ways in which a lack, or relative lack, of spontaneity can be identified.

Malcolm had started coming to me only recently.

'After the last session,' he said, 'I immediately made the two phone calls you'd encouraged me to make. I'm sure it was right and I'm glad I did. But I don't feel any better for it. Yesterday, I had a few hours off and I did nothing; I couldn't bring myself to do anything useful and I couldn't relax. It's horrible.'

'What happens on holiday?'

'Oh, no problem. When I have my two weeks off each year I just let go.' (It is typical of Malcolm that, unlike most professional people, he only manages to take two weeks off.)

'You have permission to do nothing then, haven't you?'

'Yes, that's it. Anyway I had a dream that night. The nice Mr Freud thinks we ought to talk about dreams, I believe, so perhaps it's not surprising I should have one.'

The dream was long, complicated, and interesting. At one point he had been attacked by a man and responded by beating him on the head repeatedly with a stick. I commented that it indicated the savagery that was in him.

'But it wasn't an uninhibited savagery,' he said, and made gestures in the air with his hands; these were not karate chops but had something of their precision. 'It would have been more healthy if it had been. It was very calculated, very accurate, almost intellectual. I've never hit anyone outright in my life. I would like to do so. I'd so like to do something in which I wouldn't give a damn.'

In another part of the dream there was a man of whom it was said, with admiration, 'that he had confronted his father'. This, Malcolm remarked, he himself had never done. His home had been oppressive and inhibited; sex was unimaginable; he had never been able to express himself. At this point he broke into a smile. Malcolm has an engaging, dry sense of humour but his speech is serious and thoughtful, and one has to look carefully for the fun and warmth that is in him but which only at times shows itself openly.

This description suggests that Malcolm is a weak man; but he is not. He can well stand up for himself and confront, with courage and forcefulness, anyone who does him an injustice. He felt, to me, someone to be reckoned with. So how, I wondered, were these two apparently opposite characteristics to be reconciled.

It seemed that Malcolm's spontaneity was inhibited by fears that his anger would hurt others, and that if he had allowed his feelings to emerge in childhood he would damage or destroy a family who did not deserve such retribution. But, if given permission to be himself, as on holiday or when provoked to aggression, his spontaneity could emerge. He could react, but not act.

Richard, in a sad and resigned way, saw the world as a kind of brick wall, a hard place with which there could be no negotiation. His aim in life was to adapt to it as best he could, keep a low profile, make few demands, and hope for a quiet time. He did not believe in the existence of genuine love—either his own or that of other people (the one exception to this rule was his love for his small son). In therapy it was the same. He recognized that his heart was not in it. He attended, but without much hope, always fearing that I might become fed up with him and give him the boot.

On one occasion, Richard told me that he was becoming increasingly troubled that if he continued to take time off work for his second session of the week, he might get the sack. We both thought that his fear was neurotic rather than realistic. It was, however, characteristic of him that he did not think of asking whether I could make a change of time to help the situation. I asked him if it would make any difference if we moved the session to an hour earlier.

> 'It would be a nuisance to you. It would put me under an obligation to you. I couldn't cope with that. I'd feel even more guilty than I do now.'
>
> 'Well, what about a compromise? I know it's only on certain days that it's crucial for you to be at work. Let's say, on those days we have the session early, and otherwise we have it at the usual time.'
>
> 'Yes, that would be fine if you felt OK about it.'
>
> 'Yes. I'm quite happy about it.'
>
> There was a pause, then he said: 'The only thing is, it's a quid pro quo, a negotiation, it's not just one of us being spontaneous and saying, without thought of bargaining, "We'll do this". I only want things if the other person wants them. It's like sex. I don't want sex with someone who is not being selfish and simply enjoying it.'

What seemed to me significant is that he craved the spontaneous—a relationship that was not a function of duty or sympathy and did not involve the creation of an emotional debt. I found myself thinking of a mother who gives to her child with enjoyment and who therefore is not looking for any other reward or expression of gratitude. In the everyday world—perhaps especially in our particular society, built on the sanctity of wise housekeeping—such mutual and simple delight is rare.

Richard's comments also made me think about my role as a therapist. Clearly I could not love him and devote my life to him as he does to his own child. I asked him if he thought I did gain some pleasure from being with him. 'Yes, I do, at times: when you've said something that rings true and helps; and when we've laughed together or talked about something that we've been interested in.'

Although I believe that my spontaneity, insofar as it existed and manifested itself in relation to him, was important to Richard I do not wish to imply that we dispensed with a search for the origins of his particular craving for spontaneous love. Indeed, we did not. The problem was clearly present in childhood. Robert describes his mother as someone who devoted herself to looking after the children but was unable to show open affection, to hug, kiss, or play. He remembers wishing

that he had other people as parents and wondering if his own
parents wished they had a different child. His defensive move
was to dismiss them, and with them the world, as a potential
source of love and to pretend he could manage without it.

One day he told me a dream:

> 'I was swimming in a rough, grey sea when I saw a group of
> dolphins, diving in and out of the water. They were beautiful.
> One of them came and swam beside me. I noticed that its head
> was a bit like a seal. The dolphin was very warm and friendly;
> there was some kind of communication between us. By a kind
> of magic on the dolphin's part I was able to both swim and soar
> in the air without effort. It felt marvellous.'

Richard's association to dolphins was that they were 'sensitive'. He agreed with my observation that dolphins had a
rather special meaning for many people: that they were
thought of as rather more like humans than most animals and
may have connotations of mystery and magic, in the way that
animals so often have in some cultures. 'It may sound corny,'
I said, 'but the words come to my mind "We are not alone".'

> 'Yes, I think you're right. I feel absolutely alone. You can never
>   really feel what it's like for someone else. If they're vomiting
>   you may feel sorry for them, you may remember that it's a
>   horrid experience, but you can't *feel* it.'
> 'Can't one get near enough so that we are not alone? Do we have
>   to be omniscient, like God?'
> 'I would like to believe in God. I can't believe in God and I can't
>   not believe in God. I don't think our brains are made in a way
>   that makes us able to understand these things.'
> 'Yes, I feel like that too. But does your dream mean that you long
>   to believe someone could transcend this abyss between you
>   and the world—but never *enough*? The dolphin was near. How
>   big was it?'
> 'It was very big: I couldn't put my arm round it.'
> 'Do you think it was like a mother who communicates with a
>   child before there are words?'
> 'Yes, it sounds a bit like that. But of course I don't remember.'

For most of the time Richard lies on the couch. It is his custom
to sit up about five minutes before the end of the session. He
did so at this point. He now had a view of my desk. 'Good
Lord!' he said, 'the dolphin was a bit like the seal on your

desk!' (this is a bronze model of a seal). 'So the dream has something to do with me?' I questioned.

Richard has been coming to me for a long time. He is not desperately unhappy. Sometimes I wonder if I am justified in continuing to see him, and suspect that, at least in part, I do so because I enjoy his company. The session did not throw much light upon a dilemma we both know all too well. The dream was poignant, had an emotional impact on him, and I think our discussion of it was worthwhile. But what will really help him? Will it be my ability to persuade him that his vision of the world is faulty and that he need not necessarily keep it? Do I do this by discussion? Or will it be a matter of proving sufficiently reliable and genuine in my attempt to become intimate—a feat that may best be accomplished by quite simple, spontaneous or often non-verbal means which may seem ordinary to me but, if he can believe in them, a miracle to him?

> 'You see,' Richard went on, 'I couldn't have swum like this on my own. It had to come from outside. It was like magic.'
> 'It seems to me a paradox,' I said: 'The dolphin enabled you to swim, to act, to be, spontaneous. Not your usual careful, concocted, technique of getting along in life, but your real self. Yet it came from outside. One could think of it negatively as a false, spurious self taken from something outside you, or positively, one could see the dolphin as something which simply is encouraging you and enables you to be yourself. But the dream feels positive doesn't it?'
> 'Oh yes!' Richard replied emphatically. 'It was the second of those not the first. I felt real and safe.'

At this point Richard sat up. Once again, he looked at my desk

> 'And there's your seal,' he said.
> 'Perhaps that's what all this is about. I try to make you feel safe enough to be yourself. That's what you look for in me. But it's real, not magic. It can happen.'
> 'I know it can happen for other people. But it's difficult to believe it can happen for me.'

Richard was away the following week. When he next came he lay on the couch and immediately talked of the dolphin dream again. This was an indication of how much it meant to him for he usually makes little of dreams.

'The dolphin dream has faded,' he said, 'and so has the feeling it
  brought. Now everything is an effort again. I have to make
  myself do things. I don't just do them.'
'Well, whatever the dream was about it was about spontaneity.
  Either spontaneity in you or coming from outside you.'
'But what I feel *now* seems the reality, not the other.'
'I think they're both real. The dream showed what you feel
  somewhere in yourself and what you could be.'
'Yes, that's true. But what can I do about it? I can't decide to be
  spontaneous. I can't *will* it.'
'No, I agree. But perhaps you could look at what gets in the way.
  I think you're fed up with having to make an effort to do
  everything. I think you gave up spontaneity very early and
  started to do things deliberately, almost by rote' (I think of
  Winnicott's ideas as I say this). 'I don't think you've got the
  hope that you could just *do*.'
'Sometimes I can. I just sit down and paint. But today I've been
  asked to do a painting and couldn't even begin.'
'I think you haven't got the heart to just live; there's not enough
  hope. And it's a kind of sulk. And a habit. It makes me think of
  a convalescent who gets sick and begins to think he can't be
  otherwise.'
'Yes. My father was like that.'
'I think your sense of hope is so frail that if anything doesn't
  work out the hope just goes.'
'Yes. It was like that with the therapy. I just came without
  deliberation and expected it to work.' (This is true. I mistakenly
  thought I'd have a relatively easy task with this apparently
  hopeful man.)
'And then you lost heart.'
'Yes.'
'I think you thought it was going to be much easier than you ex-
  pected.'
'I don't believe things should be so difficult.'

I was torn at this point between saying: 'Don't you realize that
life *is* hard for everyone,' or 'It is particularly hard for you because you've lost your spontaneity.' What I did say was: 'You
seem to feel alone in this. But there are lots of people who are
neurotic, and often neurotic in this way, who find they have to
gird themselves up to act. I could line up rows of them for you.'
(At this point I thought of the effort I had myself had to make
to get myself together to work today but did not say this to
him.)

'Yes, I do feel I'm the only one. But I still don't know how to
    change.'
'Do you think you need to be able to allow someone—a friend or
    even a therapist—to make an impression on this, to allow
    them to give you hope?'

In most areas of his life, Richard would be considered a lively,
open, spontaneous person. I warm to this spontaneity. It is not
unconsidered, even though it is quick. Richard does not hurt
me with his comments and does not wish to hurt me. His
spontaneity is contained within the boundaries that he has set
up between himself and me and, indeed, between himself and
the world. He has adopted a style that involves risks but risks
that have been stringently calculated and can be attached, unthinkingly, to each new situation. He is not insincere; there is
no false *bonhomie*, no sense of strain. When he gets on the
couch he tells me what he is thinking. And I believe he does so
honestly. He feels a real person to me; I feel we have a real relationship; it would seem mistaken to say that he was presenting me with a 'false self'. There does not exist an ideal state in
which we (all of us) can reveal ourselves fully. There are, at
most, moments, probably rare, when we can at least approach
this state. It would therefore be stupid to expect this of
Richard. But his sense of deep loss, despite an apparently successful life, is enough to bring him to continue to come. If his
pain were greater he might be forced to abandon his gains. But
the risks are finely balanced.

After reading this account, which he confirmed was a true
one, Richard said: 'You write beautifully'. To say this as a first
response was absolutely characteristic of him. He wasn't attempting to flatter me; he meant it. But by addressing the matter from an aesthetic point of view he avoided any impact it
might have on the state of his life and any need for action.

Shortly afterwards, however, Richard came to a session and
said: 'It's all talk. It's too easy. Why don't you just tell me to
come off it and shut up?' I thought that I had, in effect, been
trying to tell him, for a long time, that it was all talk. But I
think he had a valid point. I had never, even when stirred and
angry, quite put it in such an ordinary, direct way. 'If that happened,' he went on, 'I'd be lost. I wouldn't know what to say
. . . I'd just say I'm very unhappy.' In saying this he had now
come close to expressing the feeling of unhappiness; in terms

of Trilling's distinction[2] he had moved from sincerity to authenticity. I am ashamed that, despite my belief in ordinariness, it was *he* who had to tell *me* to act in an ordinary way.

Richard's dilemma leads us back to the question of spontaneity in the therapist, for whom the risks are also finely balanced, and inevitably so. The psychotherapist is not in the consulting room to indulge in the expression of her thoughts and feelings at random; rather, she is there to help the patient express his. She needs to listen carefully, to allow space for the other to find his own voice, an undertaking that may, at times require her to be silent and reflective. She needs to explore, patiently and carefully, the story that is being told, looking for clues that will help to build a coherent and true picture of his life and plight. In taking such a stance she is offering something that is different, if only in degree, from the kind of response that such a person may meet with in his daily life. Therapists have the time, the commitment, the setting, the experience of helping others and the relative freedom from confusing emotional bonds which may enable them to maintain a receptive attitude.

The picture of receptivity that I have drawn suggests at first sight restraint rather than spontaneity. And in some ways, this is a reasonable description. But what, unhappily, has happened is that an important element in good psychotherapy—restraint—has assumed in our minds and perhaps in our practice, such a dominance that it constitutes the accepted style and structure of work. Reticence is the norm: deviations from this approach are suspect and usually considered undisciplined. The early analysts seem, for better or worse, to have been able to achieve a relatively flexible way of working. But since Freud's papers on technique (1915–19) a rigid code of behaviour has been written into the books. The analyst should adopt a non-reactive, poised, unemotional, neutral attitude in which as little is given away as possible. This can sometimes be taken to absurd lengths. I know one analyst who believes it is wrong to smile at his patients.

Given that, to a degree, we are reticent in all our relationships it is hardly surprising that we need to deploy it in therapy. The imperfections, both in ourselves and others, may be too painful or dangerous to explore. We may have characteristics which, if given vein in therapy, would harm our patients.

If we are seducers by nature we had better restrain our sexuality in the consulting room. Moreover, the patient may be so vulnerable, so on the brink of collapse, so seductive or so potentially violent that we have to tread carefully. In doing so we are responding to a unique situation between the two people; it is not necessarily an approach to be recommended at all times for all patients and all therapists.

The idea that it is desirable to be always entirely open in therapy had led in recent years to destructive experiences in some experiential groups. A desire for privacy is not necessarily pathological and is sometimes absolutely necessary.

As Smail writes:

The official psychologies or philosophies of the twentieth century have, if anything, only served to increase the vulnerability of our subjectivity. Jungian psychology's disapproving assessment of the overdeveloped "persona", Sartrean existentialism's positive valuation of "authenticity", Freudian psychology's mistrustful vigilance for "unconscious motivation", and so on, have all done their bit to contribute to what has become the banalised craving for "sincerity", an urge to collapse the public onto private and to publicise the private by turning itself inside out. It is as if the only person we could trust, including ourselves, would be one who is completely transparent outside and indistinguishable from inside.[3]

If psychotherapeutic literature is anything to go by, most practitioners come across as rather stilted, rigid, and humourless, although we do not know whether the strict regime that is presented as a model is actually adhered to when the door is closed and no one is listening in. And if I look at the way I myself am with the people who come to me for help I am sometimes appalled by my mannerisms and orderliness. Why don't I get up and stretch my legs when I feel like doing so? Why am I so hesitant to go to the lavatory during a session even when I feel the need to? Why can't I bring a cassette player into the room and suggest we have a bit of background music? Might the patient not feel easier if I were myself sufficiently relaxed to act in this kind of way?

We cannot live without a certain amount of routine; each of us develop styles of behaviour both inside and outside the consulting room. What is significant is how defensive we are, how stereotyped in ways that impede our capacity to make most use of the relationship on offer, to allow things to happen that are not always predictable and explicable. An invisible observer witnessing the therapist sitting quietly looking at the floor would be hard pressed to say whether this was stereotyped behaviour or whether the therapist was quite spontaneously and sensitively responding to a particular patient's acute need to tell his story without interruption and without the gaze of the therapist. How can we convey the tones of voice, the gestures, the subtle nuances, the interjections, the apparent inconsequentiality of much that we do or say? How can we justify including it in what we call case-histories?

To give some flavour of the sort of communicational difficulties and potential embarrassments I have in mind I will give a simple hypothetical interchange. Someone comes in and says, 'I've got a terrible cold'. How might a therapist respond? He might say (sympathetically), 'I'm sorry' or 'Yes, it does sound bad'. Or (perhaps a little dismissively), 'Have you?' or 'There's a lot around' or 'So have I'. Or (questioning): 'What does it mean to you to have a cold?' or 'Why might you have got yourself a cold' or 'These frequent colds of yours must signify something'. Or (patiently) with silence . . . waiting. It is unlikely that he would say: 'For Christ's sake, keep away from me', but he might think it. To what degree are these responses spontaneous or reflective? One cannot be sure without knowing much more about the two people and their relationship and the beliefs of the therapist, but I would guess that we are likely to think of the silence or the questioning as reflective and the other responses as spontaneous. Yet, intuitively, there may well be reflection (if immediate and hardly conscious) in a response which is sympathetic or dismissive: we may take into account, for example, the degree to which the other person is hypochondriacal, feels alone in an unsympathetic and hostile world, or sees himself as a spreader of destructive emotions. And in the comment: 'These frequent colds must signify something' there may be an exasperated, precipitate element: the therapist might really mean: 'When on earth are you going to stop taking refuge in illness and do some proper therapy?' As for the silence: that could mean anything. I imagine most of us would find it difficult to justify saying: 'For Christ's sake keep away from me', but the possibility of having this thought has a bearing on the limits of spontaneity. I will now give an actual example of apparent spontaneity in the therapist.

I work in a flat on my own and consequently I am the one who always answers the telephone. On one occasion, however, my wife was there, and, as I was momentarily occupied she answered the telephone and then handed it to me. The call was from a woman who wanted to change a session time; she sounded flustered:

'I wondered if I'd got the right house; a woman answered the phone.'

'Yes,' I said, 'you're quite right. This is the flat. That was my lover.'

The words seemed to be out of my mouth without a thought: they were, in the everyday sense of the word, spontaneous. But, of course, they were not thoughtless. I would not have replied in such a way to every patient who rang, or, indeed to this particular patient if her frame of mind had been quite different. I think I was simply indulging in a bit of light-heartedness, but it could be argued that I had a therapeutic motive. Perhaps I wished, by joking, to reassure her that I did not feel she had invaded a private relationship. Or perhaps I wished to foster her jealous fantasies by conjuring up a lover or (perhaps even more difficult to take) suggesting that my wife was my lover. Let me hasten to say that I am not assuming that I am above the narcissistic desire to be thought a bit of a Don Juan—a desire to which those of us in our seventies are rather prone.

There is bound to be a difference between long-term and short-term therapy in our likely responses to a patient. As one gets to know a person over a length of time one can usually feel safer in speaking spontaneously. On the other hand, in short-term work, and especially in a single interview, the therapist does not have to consider the future relationship—she need not, for example, worry about the effect on the transference. And, indeed, owing to the shortage of time, she may need to take more risks than the therapist who has the opportunity to introduce ideas gradually.

It is notable that when therapist and patient meet each other unexpectedly in the course of daily life—shopping, in a café, or at a party, for example—they are usually embarrassed and at a loss as to how to behave with each other. This extreme uneasiness is, I think, a measure of their fear of being seen by the other as they really are, with their defences down. Yet, if this be so, it is a strange fact, for the rationale of psychotherapy depends on the therapist perceiving the patient as he really is, and it suggests that revelations in the consulting room are more carefully monitored than is usually thought and that each partner hides behind their respective roles.

Recently a woman said: 'Since I've been coming to you I've gradually lost confidence in myself'. I was taken aback by this, and in overall terms, I doubt if it was true. But I asked myself how this might, in some way, have occurred with someone whose therapy appeared to be going reasonably well. The most likely answer I could find—and one which made sense to her—was that her continuous belief that I was a superior person who managed his life infinitely better than she managed her own had undermined her sense of worth. If I had been able to be more openly the imperfect person who is revealed when I am more spontaneous she might have been spared the temptation to idealize me at her own expense.

The sources that influence us in most of our daily lives are of two kinds. The first is someone who is publicly proclaimed an authority or expert. Today, experts are on the increase, including those in various life-situations, such as mourning, sexual abuse, and so on. (Paradoxically, at the same time we are becoming increasingly sceptical about experts: politicians, doctors, teachers, social workers, and psychotherapists have, publicly, never had it so bad.) The second way we are influenced is when we are in the presence of someone who is genuine: when his or her statements are not routine opinions or expressions of a habitual stance (like the replies when one writes to the local member of parliament), but when they are a spontaneous product of the situation, drawn out willy-nilly, when they come from the heart, relatively innocent and free from strategy or manipulation. This kind of influence is one that is more likely to occur during the course of an intimate relationship—when the two people are open with each other—and is a function of the quality of the relationship as a whole. In psychotherapy, the latter influence would appear to be of a more durable nature than that referred to as a 'transference cure', which depends on an idealization of the expert.

How do people respond to spontaneity in the therapist? My own impression is that it is more usually with relief than dismay—relief that the helper is human, possesses idiosyncrasies and vulnerabilities, and is not totally preoccupied with pursuing a technique. I will give a brief example in which a favourable consequence appeared to be the case.

A woman who no longer came to me wrote an autobiography and sent me a copy. There was little about the therapy, but a point she made was how important it had been for her when on one occasion I had said, with some heat: 'Don't you *ever* do that again!' I felt embarrassed on reading this. But perhaps the patient's own estimate is correct. As in ordinary living, it is the overall context of the relationship that matters. If, for example, a therapist were to admit having said, in exasperation: 'Cut out the crap! I can't stand it anymore. I *won't* stand it anymore', it may be thought irresponsible or even destructive, yet the patient may be deeply grateful.

In this chapter I have used the term 'spontaneity' to indicate a quality of response that comes—insofar as this is possible—from the core of one's being rather than behaviour that has been rehearsed according to a plan, strategy, or theory. It seems likely that, being unrestrained, the spontaneous mode of being would be less of an effort. The difference is akin to that between a formal dinner party in which one feels the need to behave in an acceptable way and meeting an old friend with whom one can leave one's pretences behind. Such a meeting is not a scientific search for truth but, in some ways, there is more likely to be truth around.

References

1. Cavell. M. (1993). *The psychoanalytic mind: From Freud to philosophy*, p. 116. Harvard University Press, Cambridge, MA.
2. Trilling, L. (1972). *Sincerity and authenticity*. Oxford University Press, Oxford.
3. Smail, D. (1996). *How to survive without psychotherapy*, p. 158. Constable, London.

7

Is psychotherapy an act of goodness?

Nothing matters but faith
To what matters to the heart.
Write that down for a start.
George MacBeth

It is clear that the therapist does not do her work simply out of love; if this were so she would not claim a fee. The numerous motives, conscious and unconscious, for adopting the profession include curiosity, a wish for status, a sense of moral worth, the assuaging of loneliness, the pleasure of being an object of love, voyeurism, the possibilities for creative thought, and the enjoyment of vicarious identification. The therapist is perhaps rather like the heroine in Peter Hoeg's novel *Miss Smilla's feeling for snow*, who says:

I have a weakness for loners. Invalids, foreigners, the fat boy of the class, the ones nobody ever wants to dance with. My heart beats for them. Maybe because I know I shall forever be one of them.[1]

An additional source of potential gratification is that of power. It is the manifestation of this desire—the arrogant assumption of a superior wisdom justifying the right to interfere—that has encouraged the derisory term 'do-gooders' to be applied to the helping professions. This is an accusation that we should not dismiss lightly. As Thomas Szasz has argued,[2] the history of psychiatry is a shameful one: the ready assumption of the inferiority of the deviant, the crude and ignorant classifications of those deemed mentally ill, and the cruel treatments applied to them call to mind the persecutions of those who, in medieval times, were considered to be possessed by Satan. Psychiatry and psychotherapy, Szasz maintains, are by no means free of these coercive practices. While noting the fact that the therapist's motives may be less pure than she thinks, we need to consider whether a genuinely benevolent attitude is likely to help another in distress and the ways in which it may do so.

When two people meet for the first time there is no knowing whether they will like each other or will come in time to do so. In an ideal world, therapist and patient could choose each other; but, as things are, this can happen only to a limited extent, and even then the choice may not always be made for the right reasons. I may elect to go to a therapist who seems likely to give me an easy ride; or because I am looking for someone who conveys an impression of omnipotence; or because I am sexually attracted to her. If, however, one believes—as I do—that therapy is likely to go better if the two people feel an affinity it would be wise to put some trust in one's intuition when making a choice.

There is a paradox at the heart of psychotherapy. Although someone in distress is turning to a professional and expects the kind of dedication to the task that is the mark of a good professional, he or she usually develops a desire, often intense, for an experience of a quite different nature—an intimate, personal, and loving relationship. The crucial and agonizing question for the patient is: 'Do you put up with me because it is your professional duty to do so or do you actually care about me?' It is, I think, a legitimate question.

Freud, to his discomfort, came across the craving for love early in his career and was later to conceive it as 'positive transference': the patient's recapitulation of yearnings towards their parent. This concept can take us a long way but its explanation is limited. There are other, and simpler, explanations of the tendency for people to yearn for the love of their therapist. Whatever their childhood experience or fantasies, it is not surprising that someone should develop strong feelings towards the person to whom he has opened his heart, who offers him a quite unusual amount of concentrated attention, and who may have also give him some of the help that he so badly needs—quite apart from any sexual feelings that might be aroused in the course of intimate conversations over a long period of time. Indeed, after such exposure to the other's gaze, he might well think: 'If there is anything of worth in me at all, how cannot this person have some good feelings towards me?' In other words, given these circumstances, we might well expect that the client should want more than competent and dispassionate service performed as a duty. If the therapist were to be asked whether she really cares, what could she say? Would she even know the answer herself? (I am, for the sake of argument, leaving aside the important fact that the therapist will—to put it mildly—care for some patients more than others.)

Let us consider the kind of situation as it occurs in everyday living. What makes two people stick together? In the case of an authentic friendship they do so because they like each other more than they hate each other. Unless we are completely cynical about the matter, we would say that, leaving aside all materialistic considerations ('It's useful to have someone feed my cats when I'm away'), we gain sufficient enjoyment from his company and have sufficient concern for his well-being that we hold on. But there are limits. We may have supper with him now and again, go for walks with him, or invite him to stay for a few days. But we do not (usually) ask him to live with us. We need our freedom too badly and we have only a limited amount of tolerance for those of his habits and opinions which grate on us. We may take a risk and have a month's holiday together—which the friendship may or may not survive.

If good psychotherapy enables something akin to friendship to develop how is this possible and what is its nature? There are certain features that are favourable to such an outcome. The two people are likely to be highly motivated to make a go of the relationship. They have in common the aim of influencing the state of being of one of them—a worthwhile undertaking. The focus of the discussions are intimate. This is certainly the case with the patient, who will come to realize that a good outcome will only be achieved if he is open and honest about himself. The degree to which this is true of the therapist is more debatable. Some therapists, on principle or unwittingly, reveal much of themselves; and even those who believe in concealing their reactions are likely to feel close to someone who trustingly shows his frailty.

When two people marry in church it is customary for the clergyman to ask the congregation whether there is anyone among them who can give a good reason why the event should not take place. He would be unlikely to expect some-one to say: 'But George isn't up to it! He hasn't thought about it enough. He's not prepared himself. He's not gone to any marriage advice classes'. Maybe one day such objections will be acceptable: but not now.

In one sense, the therapist's position is different from that of the bride or groom for she will be expected to have thought about it and prepared herself. But in another sense she is much in the same boat. She has dedicated herself to do something even if love fails. And therefore she has a motive for continuing even if she hates the patient and wishes he would kill himself. She may even continue for the money; like Houseman's mercenaries, she will 'save the sum of things for pay'. To what extent the therapist carries on and behaves decently out of love, dedication, pride, guilt, money, or sheer bloody-minded doggedness we can never know for sure in an individual case. Professionalism, may, at times, be the means whereby the show stays on the road. And we can justly praise it. But, like love, professionalism is not enough, and the patient will be the first to say so. With a precision which at times can be almost uncanny he will notice the ways in which his therapist cares and does not care. And lack of belief in the genuine care of the therapist is the quickest route to loss of hope.

How does therapeutic care compare to that we show to others in life? We know that love cannot be measured, yet, in a rough and ready way, we can see when it is powerful. The most obvious example is that of a mother for her child. She will stay by him for night after night when he is seriously sick, with little thought for her own needs. If necessary, she will die for him. Even when we take account of duty, of ambivalence, of narcissistic identification, or if we invoke Darwin, we do not eliminate a phenomenon which is there before us as simply as most of the things in life that we manage to accept. This degree of love cannot easily be aroused in much of living. There are likely to be very, very few people concerning whom we would say to God, in secret, 'Take *me*; not *him*'. It would be rare for this small list to include even dearest friends and dearest patients. The patient intuitively knows this, and sometimes finds the care intolerably short of his desire; yet, paradoxically, he is getting a quality of attention for lengths of time that cannot usually be managed by those closest to him.

The prevalent belief that emotional feelings towards patients are to be deplored because they obstruct an objective assessment of their condition is an error consequent upon the separation, in philosophical thought, of reason and emotion (to which I refer elsewhere in this book). Emotion is not, of course, guaranteed to be a beautiful thing which inevitably leads to truth. Like everything else, it can be good or bad. But if we were to eschew everything in life that can potentially be bad there would be little left to live for. To permit or encourage feelings in the consulting room need not be an open invitation to intolerance or self-indulgence. Emotion does, however, carry certain dangers for the therapist's well-being. There is a threshold, which varies for one practitioner to the next, beyond which the extent of her emotional engagement with anguished people becomes too draining. But she has an answer to this: she sees her patients for limited periods and she takes holidays.

If the emphasis of the word 'professional' is placed on an attitude of dedication and responsibility it becomes closely intertwined with the concept of care, but if it is understood as a claim to a special skill or technique, as in the case of a lawyer, accountant or surgeon, the proficiency of the exercise is considered to be what matters. Let us take the case of the surgeon as an example. The surgeon is paid to undertake life-saving operations and the good that she does may well be more important to her than the money she receives. Yet, in the actual performance of her task she is not required, in a direct, interpersonal way, to behave well towards the patient, let alone love him, for the latter is unconscious of what is going on. The surgeon's ethical behaviour is concerned with applying technique to the best of her ability. If the couple were to be together when one of them is not unconscious they may loathe each other. This would be sad, but the important matter is whether or not a tumour has been successfully removed. The psychotherapist, by contrast is in no such position. The hazards she faces are of a different kind. If the surgeon's hand is shaky, the patient (mercifully) will not know. If the therapist's hand is shaky the other person will be concerned to know the reason ('Is she *that* angry with me?'). The therapist's love or hate, care or indifference, will affect the patient directly and emotionally, and will intrinsically modify the outcome of the undertaking. If the therapist does, in fact, hate her patient (i.e. experiences a continual and relentless feeling of dislike or revulsion) all, as I suggest above, is not necessarily lost. It would seem to be the worst possible scenario, one to be avoided at all costs. Yet, even in such unpropitious circumstances the therapist may manage to contain her hate, to behave decently and responsibly, and perform the equivalent of a good incision, not out of savagery but out of a wish to do an efficient piece of work on someone who is not simply a mass of flesh or a worthless entity but a human being in need.

James Fenton has described a reported interchange between Michelangelo and Giambologna:

In old age, Giambologna used to tell his friends the story of how, as a young man, a Flemish sculptor newly arrived in Rome, he made a model to his own original design, finished it *coll'alito*, "with his breath"—that is to say, with the utmost care, bringing it to the very peak of finish—and went to show it to the great Michelangelo. And Michelangelo took the model in his hands and completely destroyed it, and then remodelled it according to his way of thinking, and did so with marvellous skill, so that the outcome was quite the opposite of what the young man had done. And then Michelangelo said to Giambologna: now go and learn the art of modelling before you learn the art of finishing . . .

They must have seemed like hours, as the young sculptor watched, and the wrathful old genius, biting his lower lip, squeezed and squashed and pounded away at the model that had been so lovingly finished. And well before the new model began to emerge, and with the ostensive reason for the exercise—learn to model before you learn to finish—another point was being made: See how I crush all your ambitions and aspirations, see how feeble your work is in comparison to mine, see how presumptuous you were even to dare to cross the threshold—Thus I destroy you!

There were compensations of course, for the young Giambologna. He had walked in with an example of his juvenilia, and he left carrying a vibrant little Michelangelo. You might say that he was lucky the master had thought him worthy of the lesson, even if the lesson had to be delivered in such a devastating way. You might say this. Or you might argue that the ostensive lesson was only a pretext for the destruction of the young man's work.[3]

Fenton concludes that Giambologna does eventually benefit from Michelangelo's savage lesson. But he might not have done: he might have given up art on the spot or he might have gone home and cut his throat. If Michelangelo's harsh action was performed out of love, it was likely to be a love of art rather than love of the pupil. But, from the recipient's point of view, the master's emotional state was perhaps not of much significance: what counted was his opinion.

The psychotherapist may sometimes be faced with a situation not unlike the one described above. The difference however, is that his 'lesson' concerns the whole being of the other: the therapist is therefore more likely to consider the possibility of suicide than did Michelangelo but he still might have to take the risk.

It is understandable that a therapist who believes that she can help patients by her decency, honesty, and care may be hesitant in saying so. This, perhaps, is one of the reasons why even with the work of Ferenczi and Suttie, and the research findings on the efficacy of a caring attitude, the profession continues to marginalize love in favour of technical competence. The conviction that the cool, impersonal approach of the physical scientist is appropriate to our intimate relationships with each other is still prevalent, if not always stated overtly. A further reason why we are squeamish about the matter of care is that it cannot be easily articulated in a way that can be demonstrated with precision. Moreover, morality, in current philosophical thinking is largely considered in terms of logic as, for example, in the influential work of Rawls:[4] what is good is what is just and what is just is amenable to logical argument. This view of morality has been challenged by several writers, notably John MacMurray, Mary Midgeley, and Martha Nussbaum. While not doubting the value of the dominant stance in philosophy, Nussbaum[5] deplores the absence of deep understanding of the complexity and sheer messiness of life that, by contrast can be encapsulated in great literary art, and takes the Aristotelian view that reasoning is an insufficient means of achieving practical wisdom. This line of thought suggests to us that the psychotherapist can only perceive her patient truly if she allows herself to rely on her feelings.

Freud's own views on love have much to do with the psychoanalytic emphasis on technique. He had the utmost contempt for the Christian ethic of charity. What good will it do, he asked, to love someone? As Roazen puts it:

The egocentricity of Freud's argument has gone almost unnoticed; yet as early as before World War I, Alfred Adler had pointed out the unacceptability of Freud's attack on altruistic love (Adler came to believe that Freud's whole psychology, including the concept of the Oedipus complex, reflected the thinking characteristic of a spoiled child.) Freud, however, was unremitting in his dissection of the proposed ideal to love one's neighbour.[6]

Freud's attitude to his fellowmen—which included dividing his patients into the 'worthy' and the 'worthless'—contrasts sharply with his conviction that his work was scientifically and morally neutral. Psychoanalytic thinking comes closest to valuing the practitioner's emotion in the recognition that 'countertransference' (the feeling response of the therapist to the patient) is a good guide to what is going on in the latter. The therapist's gut reactions, however, in terms of this formulation, become a source of knowledge only of use in conjunction with the intellectual addition of self-analysis undertaken by an expert in the field. Scientific technique has crept back into the idea and unnecessarily complicated matters; emotion is still subsumed by intellect.

In a paper read to the British Psychoanalytical Society in 1960 Rycroft[7] described the treatment of a schizophrenic man who 'appeared to have abandoned every device by which human beings endeavour to make themselves interesting and acceptable to others'. There were, however, unguarded moments when this defence did not work. At the beginning of the first session 'when he lay down on my couch he immediately discovered a position in which he could without discomfort gaze at me, and then gave me one beautiful smile which permanently endeared him to me'. The phrase: 'permanently endeared him to me' is a striking one and, in the context of the time and the place, a brave one. If I remember correctly, one member of the audience, who could not believe his ears, asked Rycroft to repeat it. In view of the immense difficulties which

Rycroft endured with tenacity over the years (the patient carried a hammer in his pocket when he came to sessions) it seems that the words were not spoken lightly.

In the *Oxford companion to philosophy* references to love are meagre, to say the least, but one can find a note that,

in discussions of virtue(s) there has been much disagreement over whether conscientious adherence to duty is morally preferable to "natural" motivations like compassion or love as a basis for actions.[8]

Bernard William's observations on the pursuit of virtuous behaviour are perhaps relevant to his question. He comments that,

the cultivation of the virtues has something suspect about it, of priggishness or self-deception.[9]

This kind of reflection, he believes, inclines towards thinking about,

the way in which others might describe or comment on the way in which you think about your actions, and if that represents the essential content of your deliberations, it really does seem a misdirection of the ethical attention.

The picture that Williams conjures up has, unhappily, the ring of truth, but it does not include the possibility that we may try to be good for the sake of someone else's well-being (i.e. that the pursuit of virtue can be based on love).

The suggestion that personal caring tends to be relegated to the sidelines in philosophy and psychology receives support from a study by Carol Gilligan on the moral beliefs of women.[10] Gilligan found that, in contrast to the received philosophical view of morality (propounded, as she emphasizes, by men) which is founded on duty, justice, autonomy, and abstraction, women place more emphasis on the value of caring and relationships. It is not a surprising finding for it is our daily observation that this is the case. Gilligan uses her findings to challenge the accepted view not only of what is good moral behaviour but what should be included in the concept of morality itself. She not only strikes a blow both for feminism (showing that Kohlberg's[11] influential attribution of inadequacy in the female sense of morality is based on false premises), but asks us to take a new look at traditional moral philosophy. One of the attractions of Gilligan's ideas are that they take us away from the abstractions of Kantian thinking on morality and face us with the particularities of living as a particular person in relation to others sharing a common culture—an emphasis that has earlier been made by Mac-Intyre.[12] It is this aspect of Gilligan's work that is the focus of its exposition by Hekman.[13] Although a passionate supporter of Gilligan, with whom she identifies as a fellow feminist, Hekman shows that these ideas, in doctrinal forms, are to be found in the writings of many others, including Iris Murdoch, Simone Weil, and Michael Oakeshott. What is required, she believes, is a new paradigm for morality, in which the disembodied, abstract self gives place to a concept of morality that exists and shows itself in relation to others. It is, however, in the thoughts of another philosopher influenced by Gilligan, Annette Baier, that the issues of care, trust, and love, so central to the theme of this chapter, are more directly addressed.

Baier[14] maintains that women's moral theory, expressive of their insights and concerns, would be an 'ethics of love'. This is to be contrasted with men's theories, which are based on obligation. Much of her argument derives from the belief that children are best reared if their parents are loving, and that no account of morality which ignores this fact and focuses on the concepts of obligation and justice in the making of a good society can therefore be adequate:

Undoubtedly some important part of morality does depend in part on a system of threats and bribes, at least for its survival in difficult conditions when normal goodwill and normally virtuous dispositions may be insufficient to motivate the conduct required for the preservation and justice of the moral network for relationships. But equally undoubtedly life will be nasty, emotionally poor, and worse than brutish (even if longer), if that is all morality is, or even if that coercive structure of morality is regarded as the backbone, rather than as an available crutch, should the main support fail.[15]

The feminist issues expressed here are not directly relevant to the matter under discussion and there are many who would question the implication that women are morally superior to men, but the psychotherapist reading Baier will, I believe, be likely to find echoes in his or her heart when thinking about their work. Although patients are not children (indeed, it would be grotesquely patronizing to think so) they are, in view of their vulnerability to the therapist's power, in a position not unlike that of the child and therefore need, in some ways, the kind of emotional responses necessary to the rearing of children.

The distinction between professional care and personal care would appear to be a particular form of the distinction between love and duty which has troubled philosophers throughout history. In the modern age, virtue is seen as a conscientious and effortful attempt to act in an ethical way: to be good is to be dutiful. And this is how Freud saw it, although he put the matter in very different terms. For Freud love was not primary. A person 'loved' because the object of love is useful, either sexually or in other ways. It is not surprising, therefore, that Freud derived his concept of social ethics from factors other than love. Forrester, with customary rigour, erudition, and apt quotation, shows the degree to which Freud, like Nietzsche, believed that a sense of justice derives from envy.[16] The envious person says, in effect: 'If I can't have it nobody else shall'. Forrester writes:

We may have become able to accept a base genealogy for religion and Christian morality; at the very least, the Freudian and Nietzschian critiques have habituated us to the idea that humility and brotherly love may be based on fear and resentment. But how relaxed are we about seeing our sense of justice based on envy? It seems we are now accustomed to God being dead, but would be reluctant to admit that social justice died from similar causes.[17]

Yes, we might well be reluctant—but an argument based on our reluctance to accept a suggestion does not necessarily carry the day. Psychotherapists and those influenced by Freud's scepticism may well be more embarrassed to admit a belief in love and virtue (and a connection between the two) than to claim affinity with Freud's tough-minded and stoical approach.

There are some areas where common sense fails us. The sun, it seems, does not encircle the earth. But for most areas in our lives, common sense is not to be dismissed, and the philosophical arguments that contradict it should be viewed with caution. We may do well to assert, with Bernard Williams,[9] that it is a corruption of language to deny the moral value of a disposition (love) which, as our daily experience shows us, is an important element in achieving good. To affirm the efficacy of goodness does not involve us in a denial of the fact that goodness can itself be tainted or used for corrupt purposes.

If we take seriously the idea that the therapist's goodness or lack of it is a central factor in the undertaking we will need to make a significant change in psychotherapeutic theory. The term 'paradigm shift' is perhaps too easily bandied about at present but we are, I believe, dealing with something of that order, for we are in the realm of the moral rather than that of science, and we stand or fall by our practical wisdom rather than our technique. What is not included in the contemporary view of therapy is the idea that cognitive understanding, although central to any useful communication between two people in almost any circumstances, does not necessarily constitute the primary aim when therapist and patient meet in order to bring about something good between them: the wish to do good to each other, and the authenticity of that wish, is perhaps at least of comparable importance; and the perceptions by each partner of this authenticity may be as useful in improving matters as anything else that occurs.

To understand other people is an ordinary part of living. We all attempt, with varying degrees of success, to do it, and we do not regard this achievement as a special accomplishment requiring specialized training at institutions set up for the purpose (at least, not until the advent of psychotherapy). But, because of the immense respect for cognitive functioning in professional circles—and, indeed, among much of the lay population—it does not seem strange to most people in our society to believe that we can improve understanding primarily by using special methods of observation and making new theoretical formulations. In the case of the wish to do good, however, the matter is quite different. There are no psychotherapeutic organizations, as far as I know, that base their theory, practice, and teaching on ways in which a therapist may improve his or her urges to do good. To attempt to set up such an organization—or to include in one's programme seminars designed to enhance a psychotherapist's desire to do good—would, I think, be an embarrassing thing to do. We leave that to religion, and to get mixed up with that sort of thing (except, following Freud, to analyse it) would be considered scientifically disreputable. However, in the same way that fruitful inroads have been made with the ordinary capacity to understand people, it is possible that a comparable attempt could be made in the context of psychotherapy to

improve someone's desire and capacity to be good, in a favourable setting, to a person in distress. In a democracy there is no
one who has the authority to teach adults how to live. Consequently, insofar as psychotherapy is centred on this question,
there is no one who can teach how to practise psychotherapy.
Recognizing the degree to which it is a moral undertaking
leaves a huge hiatus in any programme designed to instruct a
student of psychotherapy. But, perhaps something can be
learnt. Talking with people who have tried to help those in distress can give some understanding of the problems involved,
provided such knowledge is not confused and corrupted by a
failure to recognize the limitations of any attempt to formulate
the undertaking in a systematic way.

A colleague of mine was going through a difficult period
with his practice. There was a dearth of referrals and his finan-
cial problems were mounting. The next time I saw him he was
buoyant, for referrals had come his way and his money troubles were, at least for the moment, at an end. 'But I soon realized,' he said, 'that there was more to it than the money.' I
expected him to talk about a renewed sense of work as a professional and breadwinner, and so on. But he had something
different in mind. 'I felt enriched and excited by the people just
being in the room. They were unknown and I was going to get
to know them. It felt like an adventure.'

'Like two people starting out on a journey together?' I
asked. 'Yes,' he said: 'With no maps.'

There was something about his attitude that put me in mind
of the excited feeling when two people meet who sense they
might become friends or lovers. But my colleague was no
starry-eyed rookie (contrary to a widespread public belief,
even experienced psychotherapists can have their lean times)
and he did not anticipate eternal bliss.

I cannot think of an adequate way of conceiving his
response and he did not offer one. It is not enough to say it was
intellectual excitement, or love, or compassion, or a need to
heal or the assuaging of loneliness. It expressed an effortless
enthusiastic wish to be intimately engaged with someone in
the pursuit of an exciting and slightly frightening journey towards a desirable end. And it seemed to me to be an act that
was good. It may well be that later on—on occasions when he
was feeling tired or ill or when the patient is sadistically

tormenting him, that an act of will would be required in which he responds to a sense of duty or honour and obeys something akin to the Christian ethic, the Kantian imperative or the Freudian super-ego. But this would be a different kind of goodness.

References

1. Hoeg. P. (1993). *Miss Smilla's feeling for snow*, p. 40. (trans. F. David). Harvill, London.
2. Szasz, T. (1970). *The manufacture of madness*. Harper & Row, New York.
3. Fenton, J. (1995). A lesson from Michelangelo. *New York Review of Books*, 23 March.
4. Rawls, J. (1971). *A theory of social justice*. Harvard University Press, Cambridge, MA.
5. Nussbaum, M. (1990). *Love's knowledge: Essays on philosophy and literature*. Oxford University Press.
6. Roazen, P. (1991). Nietzsche and Freud. *Psychohistory Review*, Spring, 340.
7. Rycroft. C. (1987). On the defensive function of schizophrenic thinking and delusion-formation. *Imagination and reality*, p. 84. Hogarth, London.
8. Honderich, T. (ed.) (1995). *Oxford companion to philosophy*, p. 901. Oxford University Press.
9. Williams, B. (1985). *Ethics and the limits of philosophy*, p. 10. Fontana, London.
10. Gilligan, C. (1982). *In a different voice: Psychological theory and women's development*. Harvard University Press, Cambridge, MA.
11. Kohlberg, L. (1981). *The philosophy of moral development*. Harper & Row, San Francisco.
12. MacIntyre, A. (1985). *After virtue: A study in moral theory*. Duckworth, London.
13. Hekman, S. J. (1995). *Moral voices, moral selves: Carol Gilligan and feminist moral theory*. Polity Press, Oxford.
14. Baier, A. (1994). *Moral prejudices*. Harvard University Press, Cambridge, MA.
15. Ibid., p. 14.
16. Forrester, J. (1997). *Dispatches from the Freud wars: Psychoanalysis and its passions*. Harvard University Press, Cambridge, MA.
17. Ibid., pp. 42, 43.

8

Goodness, shame, and autonomy

He came home. Said nothing.
It was clear, though, that something had gone wrong.
He lay down fully dressed.
Pulled the blanket over his head.
Tucked up his knees.
He's nearly forty, but not at the moment.
He exists just as he did inside his mother's womb,
clad in seven walls of skin, in sheltered darkness.
Tomorrow he'll give a lecture
on homeostasis in megagalactic cosmonautics.
For now, though, he has curled up and gone to sleep.

Wislawa Szymborska

A middle-aged man, John, was recalling his wedding many years ago. The reception was going well, speeches were made, photographs taken, and everyone was congratulatory, as he moved around among the guests. When he approached a group of four or five people, one of them, a tough, bluff, outspoken man said, 'Why've you come here? *We* don't want to talk to you.' Although spoken dead pan it was presumably said as a joke. But John was devastated and had no response. Suddenly the whole occasion seemed a sham. He felt that he had merely been performing and, although the others had taken him at his face value, this man had seen him as the worthless creature he was; he had been revealed publicly in all his wretched nakedness.

This intense feeling of shame was not brought about by any particular action of John's. He was simply behaving in his accustomed style in a social situation. The shame derived from the recognition that his life was not as good as he tried to believe, and tried to persuade others to believe, and the sudden fear that this deception was recognized publicly.

John was a person who took responsibility for his life; he did not, for example, excuse himself with the thought, 'I have a neurosis and cannot help being this way'. His sense of shame engendered a wish to change and was therefore a potential source of growth and a help to a therapist. But shame is not necessarily a useful feeling. It can be paralysing and discouraging. If someone comes to me who feels wretched, worthless, and ashamed, it may be best to do all I can to counteract this feeling, to show him, by my demeanour and comments, that I respect him as a person who is not unworthy. It would, however, be unwise to take this approach too far and to pretend that his limitations and faults were not real and a cause for concern. Recently, in discussion with someone who was almost paralysed by a sense of shame we found ourselves wondering about the difference between chiding and encouraging. Both attitudes presuppose that an effort to change is necessary but whereas the word 'chiding' implies that the person is not already doing their best, encouraging raises the possibility that something hitherto unimaginable is within their grasp.

We consult a doctor, a psychiatrist, or a psychotherapist because we feel that something is wrong with us. Insofar as he is influenced by the traditional medical model the psychotherapist will, in his turn, also focus on what is wrong; he may make a diagnosis or look for defensive mechanisms. But this is not necessarily the best thing to do to someone who is already ashamed of themselves. It may be more useful to dwell on what is right, to acknowledge and celebrate the courage and ingenuity by which the patient has managed to carve out a life in the face of innate limitations and adverse experience. Contemporary teaching of psychotherapy tends to fail the student by steering him towards the negative.

The concept of responsibility is central to this matter. To what extent can those in despair do something about their

plight? This is a variable we can only understand intuitively.
The patient of whom I have just spoken could not, I believe,
have emerged from the session and taken a train to Land's
End, but it is within the realms of possibility that instead of re-
turning home to stare at the wall all day he could, for example,
pick up a pen and write something, possibly a letter. I likened
his position to the prisoner in solitary confinement who might
choose to write rather than slowly die even if he had little belief that the writing was valuable. I know that I chose writing
because, occasionally, I do it as a means to get myself out of a
bad state of mind; another therapist would, no doubt, have
found a different way of making the point.

The question of responsibility for our actions is the bane and
fascination of philosophers, psychologists, and psychoanalysts.
Szasz[1] challenges the 'myth' that people are not responsible
for their neurotic symptoms but he makes the mistake, as did
Freud, of building a theory that is too dependent on one particular kind of behaviour, namely, hysterical. One way of putting the dilemma is to say that autonomous action is a function
of the degree to which we have escaped our conditioning.

Another man, Richard, said to me, 'I don't have a problem
about what is best for others to do. I simply say, "I think you
should do such and such". And if they make a mess of things I
don't write them off. But when it comes to me I feel I've only
one way to live and that's to please my mother. I don't mean
how she is now (although that's there a bit, too) but how she
was. I feel a terrible weight of responsibility to make her
happy.'

This competent man was describing the sort of feeling that
haunts so many who seek help from therapists. He has learnt
from his mother how he should live and his own experience
and intelligence make no impact on the lesson. 'Everyone', he
says, 'is my mother.' He is describing the phenomenon that
Freud formulated as the super-ego (a concept later elaborated
to include the projection of the child's aggression in forming
such a hard taskmaster). Richard would, I think, be called a
good man. 'But I am a fake', he says, 'I'm not really engaged,
in my heart, with life. I get along. I avoid trouble.'

What are we to think of the nature of Richard's goodness?
This is not a man whose concealed hate permeates the air
around him and whose brittle smile warns us to keep our

distance, but someone who is sufficiently integrated and adjusted to earn the liking and respect of others. Are we to dismiss his way of being as a mere performance, the manifestation of what Winnicott refers to as a 'false self'?

I think not; the distinction between 'true' and 'false self' is a useful one in practice but does not adequately encompass the complexity of the mind. Let me put the question in a different way: How do we compare a moral sense that has been taught and unthinkingly accepted with one gained through wide experience of life and is the product of individual thought? The distinction is far from clear; none of us creates our own moral system, indeed, in postmodernist thought, each one of us is in total thrall to the culture in which we happen to be born. But most readers will, I think, accept that in practice, both in and out of the consulting room, there is a significant difference in the degree with which people have emancipated themselves from a narrow system of thought learnt in childhood.

A moral stance, it would seem, is only possible if it is not a function of the super-ego. Cavell very clearly distinguishes between refraining from doing something because one does not want to feel guilty or because such action threatens something or someone that one values. Freud, she maintains, views morality 'as a fancy name for self-interest':

While the super-ego may explain various neurotic forms of self-punishment, precisely what it doesn't explain, nor even make room for, is the moral point of view, which demands just what Freud's reduction of all interests to self-interest won't allow: valuing something because one holds it to be valuable in itself.[2]

The super-ego, then, is a negative force. It may drive us to do good but only out of fear. Indeed, it is difficult to argue convincingly against the proposition that any altruistic acts are performed in order to rid oneself of a sense of guilt and, consequently, are acts of self-interest. We may, therefore, do better to look beyond the sense of guilt in our search for the origins of our moral sense.

Bernard Williams criticizes the importance given to guilt as a source of moral behaviour. Guilt, he maintains, is a narrower concept than shame; the latter is concerned with the kind of beings we are and the failings or inadequacies that lead us to do harm.

To the modern consciousness, guilt seems a more transparent moral emotion than shame. It may seem so, but that is only because, as it presents itself, it is more isolated than shame is from other elements of ones self-image, the rest of ones desires and needs, and because it leaves out a lot even of ones ethical consciousness. It can direct one towards those who have been wronged or damaged, and demand reparation in the name, simply, of what has happened to them. But it cannot by itself help one to understand one's relations to those happenings, or to rebuild the self that has done these things and the world in which that self has to live. Only shame can do that, because it embodies conceptions of what one is and of how one is related to others.[3]

It is our misconception of the nature of shame that has led us to underestimate the morality of the Greeks. In a brilliant discussion of Greek literature, Williams shows that the concept had a much deeper resonance than the fear of public exposure. Shame, for the Greeks, was not,

just a matter of being seen, but of being seen by an observer with a certain view. Indeed, the view taken by the observer need not itself be critical: people can be ashamed of being admired by the wrong audience in the wrong way. Equally, they need not be ashamed of being poorly viewed, if the view is that of an observer for whom they feel contempt.[4]

The observing other is 'conceived as one whose reactions I would respect; equally, he is conceived as one who would respect those same reactions if they were appropriately directed at him'. Understood in this way, the Greek view of shame can illuminate our own understanding the concept:

The ethical work that shame did in the ancient world was applied to some values that we do not share, and we also recognise the separate existence of guilt. But shame continues to work for us, as it worked for the Greeks, in essential ways. By giving through the emotions a sense of who one is and of what one hopes to be, it mediates between act, character, and consequence, and also between ethical demands and the rest of life. Whatever it is working on, it requires an internalised other, who is not designated merely as a representative of an independently identified social group, and whose reactions the agent can respect. At the same time, this figure does not merely shrink into a hanger for those same values but embodies intimations of a genuine social reality—in particular, of how it will be for ones life with others if one acts in one way rather than another. This was in substance already the ethical psychology even of the archaic Greeks, and, despite the modern isolation of guilt, it forms a substantial part of our own.[5]

Thus, the positive change which can come about as a consequence of shame is neither a blind acceptance of another's dogma nor an isolated decision which takes no consideration of the views of others.

The feelings of shame and guilt are so interwoven that it is difficult to separate them experientially; but many attempts have been made to define the difference theoretically. Most thinkers conceive shame in a similar way to Williams: the appropriate feeling when something occurs to reveal that one is less a person than one thought and that others had thought. One's whole being is exposed and under threat. Guilt, on the other hand, refers to an act which harms others, for which anger and punishment might reasonably be expected, but for which reparation is possible. Jacoby observes that,

shame is often felt as a deeper injury than guilt and that guilt may therefore be used as a defence against shame. For example, if one is rejected by a lover it may be less painful to search for one's mistakes or offensive actions than to accept that one was simply not attractive or sexy enough.[6]

The shamed person has to repair himself in order to be, in some way or in some degree, a different person—one who no longer does such things. It is therefore central to the experience of psychotherapy: by exposing himself to the possibility, even likelihood, of shame, the patient asks for compassion and for help to change.

It would seem from this line of thought that the psychotherapist's role is not only to interpret the patient's repressed shortcomings and destructive urges but to take on the function of the 'respected other', who need not be idealized, but who, in an ordinary way, is seen as a decent person whose values are not easily cast aside and from whom one would wish to have reciprocal respect. The 'respected other' is there in the room, willing to listen and converse, and an opportunity is provided for a more rigorous and open revelation of thoughts and feelings than can easily be obtained in other areas in life. Williams' argument helps us to see even more clearly the moral nature of a therapeutic endeavour, the closeness between life in the consulting room and outside it, and the capacity of ordinary language to articulate moral ideas which are often inadequately expressed in psychotherapeutic theory.

There are many who live apparently competent lives and are respected by their fellows yet feel a fraud, who stride about the world with apparent purpose, yet, behind the façade are like frightened rabbits unable to emerge from their holes in the ground, believing that by some trick they have deceived everybody. This deception may give some comfort, but the sense of shame survives their successful performance only too easily and can cripple them emotionally. For those who are in this sort of predicament the respect of a therapist can mean a lot. But the sense of shame can sometimes be formidably durable even in the face of the depth of understanding that may be reached. Perhaps it is wise to recognize that shame is, to an extent, a natural state of being. It is a smug person who can look back on his life with complacency. And I am presumably not alone in warming to those who, without a narcissistic demonstration of virtuous self-revelation, can admit to shame.

I will now return to Richard. On another occasion he told me about a friend for whom he had enormous admiration. She was beautiful, intelligent and, above all, a lively, spontaneous, and warm person. What now shocked him was that, on discovering that she had been overtaken by a misfortune and was wretchedly unhappy, he felt a surge of relief and comfort.

> 'I don't really feel concerned,' he said: 'It's the feeling of comfort that is uppermost. I'm ashamed of this.'
> 'It's a human feeling, unhappily,' I replied. 'Perhaps only a saint is without envy. But I agree with you, it is shameful.'
> 'I imagine that other people don't feel like this—that when they express sympathy they mean it. *You* are sympathetic to people in trouble or you wouldn't be doing this work.'
> The less commendable reasons why I practise psychotherapy quickly flitted across my mind, but I said: 'There's a contradiction here. You say I am sympathetic to patients. Yet, in the past you've often said to me that you believe I don't give a bugger about you, that it's part of my technique to pretend that I do.' Richard laughed. 'Yes, that's true. I believe you do feel it for your other patients, not me.'
> 'Well, perhaps that may be true. Perhaps I do.'
> Richard is clearly abashed. He was not expecting this.
> I went on: 'But it may be right. And if there's something in it, it

could be because you don't provoke my sympathy. There are
people who come into this room who are so manifestly in
anguish that I can't help but feel sympathy for them. But you
don't give me that feeling. You're contained. I hear what you
say but I don't get the impact of it.'
'That's absolutely true. I know what you mean.'
'For example, when I said earlier on "It's shameful to feel that", I
found myself thinking, "But maybe Richard doesn't know that.
Maybe he doesn't really feel ashamed. Perhaps I should have
said: "You ought to be more bloody ashamed than you are".'
'Probably, but the comfort I get is so important it outweighs the
shame.'

I think that Richard obtained relief from shame from witnessing his friend's unhappy state because of the appalling weight
of having to pretend that he is in better shape than he feels. In
this sense he wants to be normal, and the distress of someone
else lowers, if only temporarily, his estimation of the state of
normality: life, he then thinks, can be too much for others too,
even the best of them. But although the therapeutic aim must
be to give him a greater sense of worth, it would need to be an
authentic sense; and to achieve this will require him to accept
that some of his thoughts and actions are really shameful. To
put the matter another way: Richard is confused between appropriate and inappropriate shame. Because he feels so unfit
for this world he finds it difficult to confront the full significance of his moral failings. In this session we had talked about
his badness. At the end, he told me that he could not come the
following week. He had taken on a daunting and very un-
pleasant task in order to help someone in trouble. I noted, to
myself, that he had not complained about this task during the
session, nor even referred to it. I was impressed by this and I
said: 'A guy who does this is not a bad guy.' As he left, he said
warmly, 'Thank you very much. It's good to have it appreci-
ated.'

Reflecting on the above I notice that at one point, presumably in an attempt to help Richard to see his shameful thought
in the context of human nature rather than an uniquely evil
tendency, I had said: 'It's a human feeling, unhappily'. I recognize that to say this may appear to condone the act, but I think
that this can be avoided by making one's position clear. I did
not mean to excuse bad behaviour. What I wanted to convey

was the thought that what he did was shameful, but that he is not uniquely shameful.

As an illustration of the sensitive balance between responsibility and shame I will quote the words of a woman who I shall call Emily.

I am not coping. I manage my work, just, but little else and inside I'm a mess. I simply can't do what most people seem able to do. They go out and they talk to people and busy themselves. But I get exhausted. If I go out to a dinner party I'm finished in an hour or two and want to go home, but all the others are only just beginning. I feel I'm "highly strung" as they liked to call it. I've always been. I can't stand much inflow, much stimulation. I get muddled. I long to leave and be by myself. But it's not that I want to be alone. Not at all. It's just that I can't take it. The best for me is being with the one or two people who I feel I am comfortable with. It gets worse as I get older. God knows what I'll be like when I'm seventy. I'll be paralytic. I envy women who can happily lead a quiet life at home.

But, for Emily, a quiet life at home would not only be lonely; it would be shameful. There are two factors at work here. First, although Emily says she envies the woman at home who is contented, this is not quite the case. The ideal she has set herself is the person who mixes well socially. The understanding she has gained during therapy is better than most of those who come to see me, and if I were to write a 'case-history' she would be a tempting choice. But despite the increased strength she has gained over the years her social life is still limited by lack of inner ease and the consequent fatigue. Can she help this, I wonder? Can we hope to alter it? Are we chasing an unrealistic explanation for the kind of person she inevitably is? I suggested to her that perhaps this is the stuff of which she is made, that she is, perhaps, by nature, sensitive and finely tuned, a state which has pluses and minuses. She was immediately relieved by this suggestion.

It is perhaps significant that in childhood Emily had an imaginary companion, taken from a character in one of her story books, who, like her, was 'oversensitive' and something of a misfit, yet whom she readily accepted as admirable despite having this attribute. Emily was able to see how easily this explanation could be used defensively; nevertheless, it enabled her to feel less ashamed of her incapacity to do certain things about which the majority of her friends seemed to have no trouble. The inabilities were still present, and she wished they were not, but, insofar as my suggestion rang true, it enabled her to feel less of a coward. I found myself wondering about the extent to which psychotherapists, who are so orientated to weeding out defences against action, may add to the patient's sense of shame over his or her inability to match society's ideal of someone who is socially at ease. For those who, being in a worse state than Emily, see themselves as a wretched, shrivelled inadequate thing, worthless to themselves and others, the question of whether or not they are responsible for their condition seems less pressing: they are as they are, for whatever reason, and the shame and misery are unbearable. In this state of mind the person craves to be 'normal' (a lesser aim than the wish to be ordinary, in the sense that I use the word in this book), to be able to get through the day without attracting pity, scorn, disgust, or contempt, and without disappointing, hurting, or embarrassing others. The task for the therapist in this case is to seize on anything, from whatever source, that will give the person the beginnings of hope. The question of their autonomy—the degree to which they can choose to change their state—cannot always be confronted directly, although it remains a perpetual challenge to our understanding and response.

References

1. Szasz, T. (1961). *The myth of mental illness.* Harper & Row, New York.
2. Cavell, M. (1993). *The psychoanalystic mind: From Freud to philosophy*, p. 217. Harvard University Press, Cambridge, MA.
3. Williams, B. (1993). *Shame and necessity*, p. 94. University of California Press, Berkeley, CA.
4. Ibid., p. 82.
5. Ibid., p. 102.
6. Jacoby, M. (1994). *Shame and the origins of self-esteem, a Jungian approach.* Routledge, London.

9

The hazards of moral judgement in psychotherapy

Speak then to me who neither needs nor fears your favours or your hate.

William Shakespeare

One of the many predicaments in life is that of making a judgement between one's own view and that of others. We are presented with this problem at almost every hour of every day. The issue involved may be a mundane matter but the decision we make will be influenced by our sense of worth and our confidence in our own perception of things; we are, moreover, often genuinely confused as to what is morally the better thing. Debate about human nature does not seem to come up with any clear answer about the motives for our judgements; whereas it is often claimed that we are egotistical beings, out to get our way at all costs, and to believe what it suits us to believe, there is plenty of evidence to show that we tend to be amazingly suggestible and conformist. Perhaps the most that can be said with any assurance is that good judgement is a manifestation of that elusive quality, wisdom.

In a therapeutic situation we have two people, each with their own views on living and each with a nervous desire to preserve those views upon which their sense of identity rests. Each is vulnerable; each has power; but each is in a different position. The therapist proclaims his ability to help and usually has a theory as to how this is best done. If the undertaking goes badly he is vulnerable to feelings of failure and suffers a blow to his professional pride and theoretical beliefs. The patient on the other hand, has both more, and less, to lose. His sense of worth is probably already at a low ebb, his need may be desperate, he may feel that the therapist is his last chance of maintaining or regaining a manageable life, but he is not burdened with the sense of professional responsibility, as is his helper. Both of them, therefore, are aware of a need to tread carefully. The therapist has to bring to bear all his sensitivity, patience, and tolerance in order to allow the patient to reveal himself. In times of crisis what he does or says may make the difference between suicide or not. The patient has the problem of whether to trust. He is in the hands of someone of status who appears to know what he is doing—but what he is doing may seem very strange. If the patient goes along with the procedure it may prove disastrous, but if he revolts he may lose all chance of whatever hope the therapist may be able to engender.

Traditionally, power and responsibility is weighted in favour of the professional. If things go wrong (if, for example, the two people have sex together) the authorities will come down heavily against him. On the other hand, the patient can also wield power (he can seduce, manipulate, and so on) and therefore he shares the responsibility. Indeed, it would be invidious to assume that he is not accountable for his behaviour.

One of the paradoxes of the classical psychoanalytic set-up is that the patient is encouraged, implicitly or explicitly, to co-operate in the venture by surrendering responsibility. 'You can say what you like, and, provided you do no significant physical harm to my body and goods, you can do what you like.' But this forbearance, if carried beyond a certain degree, may undermine the patient's sense of his own solidity and capacity to influence the world; he is not taken seriously. It would, perhaps, seem more useful and more realistic to recognize that there are two comparable people in the room, both of whom can influence the other for good and ill and both of whom have responsibility, in the eyes of God, for the other's well-being. To put it another way: the difficulty of judging a moral situation between two people in ordinary life has the same inherent qualities as that between therapist and patient.

Therapy has its own peculiar characteristics but so do other situations in society (e.g. marriage). Factors of status and power
and even law are always present and have to be dealt with.
Those of us who believe in justice and what Margolit[1] refers to
as a 'decent society' will support the view of equality of voice
in personal matters (e.g. marriage or psychotherapy) and will
argue against a disparity of responsibility. The particular obli-
gations of the two people may, however, vary from time to
time. In any circumstances, the specific liabilities that people
have towards each other are difficult to fathom, but if one of
them makes the case that his actions are justified by a particular technique the difficulty is immeasurably compounded.

On an unusually hot afternoon I had the window of my
consulting room wide open. My flat is in a quiet area; the room
is not overlooked and any sounds from outside are minimal.
Bettina came in and commented, as she lay on the couch, that
the open window made her feel uncomfortably exposed to the
outside world. Such uneasiness is not uncharacteristic of her:
she occasionally covers herself with a rug even when it is
warm. We discussed the meaning of her desire to feel enclosed
and safe. I did not, however, close the window. Later in the
session, at a point when Bettina was complaining that I practised with a rigid and ungiving psychoanalytic orthodoxy, she
again brought up the question of the window.

> 'You don't give an inch, do you? Why do you let me feel uncom-
> fortable like this? Why don't you shut the window?'
> I said: 'We could compromise, couldn't we? Surely two grown
> adults could sort out this between them? What if we kept the
> window open and drew the curtains? Then you would feel
> more enclosed and I wouldn't die of heat? Would that be OK?'
> 'Yes, I think it would.'

I drew the curtains. She thanked me. And we continued the
session.

When Bettina came for the next session the weather was
still unduly hot and we made the same arrangement over the
window. However, she became very angry with me, maintaining that, because she had never experienced understanding in
early childhood nothing would now help but someone who
would care sufficiently about her to perceive her needs. 'If you
had really understood how awful I felt exposed by the window
last time,' she said, 'you would have closed it straight away.'

One way of looking at this interchange is to consider the distribution of power in the room and the ethical considerations intrinsic to the power relation. We both have wishes and justifiable claims. I want to work in reasonable comfort and could claim that when conditions are unsuitable I will work less well. Bettina has a comparable wish for her own comfort and may believe, perhaps with justification, that her psychological need for a particular kind of therapeutic response is more important than a bit of discomfort to me. If, indeed, it were really the case then I should surely put her needs first. But can I be certain of this? Moreover, what happens to me is not only important to me but is important to her. I do not simply mean my physical or emotional well-being (for I am not, in this case, likely to die of the heat) but the emotional significance of her effect on me. In the real world—which is the world I am encouraging her to live in—people affect each other in such a way that the rights and wrongs of what they do have to be addressed. To leave out such ethical considerations is to take the patient into a very strange world. There would have to be a very good reason indeed for doing so: it would be justifiable only if her recovery depended on presenting her with the near fulfilment of an omnipotent wish. If, in fact, the ethics of the case permitted no rights to the therapist other than responding to the patient's requirements at whatever cost to himself, his family, and his other clients, it is difficult to assess who would be most endangered by such a course of action. The most sensible way to approach the kind of situation I have described would seem to be to take into consideration both the inner disturbance which Bettina brings and the real consequences of her wishes, and to respond to the situation in its uniqueness.

In the following session, Bettina returned to the matter of her absolute need of an immediate and empathic response to something very primitive in her. Without this response life meant nothing; she might as well kill herself. She seemed to have forgiven me for the lack of the 'needed' response over the window, but claimed that I was stubborn. Her description of her need was made in an emotional and convincing way and I felt painfully moved by it.

During the course of the session Bettina spoke of her mother, who is now sick and old. Even as a child, however, she felt her mother to be very needy, frightened, and clinging, and

Bettina herself felt a desperate urge to respond to this need, an incapacity to meet it, and, at times a ruthless wish to preserve herself at all costs. It seemed to us unclear whether the demand that Bettina brought to me was an expression of her authentic self or an introjection of her mother's plight.

I said that perhaps I felt towards her as she did to her mother, that when she said to me, 'I really cared about my mother most of the time but sometimes I felt hard and needed to preserve myself.' This was what I was now experiencing myself.

> 'Is that what you do feel?'
> 'Yes, I do care about you and try to help you, but sometimes I probably do become stubborn. I believe in looking after myself.'
> 'I know you do! But are my demands all that impossible?'
> 'I'm not sure how much they are simply unreasonable or how much you ask of me things that I personally cannot give.'
> 'What are the unreasonable things? Tell me. I think it would help me to know.'

After pausing to think I said: 'You take me to task for not welcoming you with open arms and a smile. Even if that were the right thing to do I still couldn't do it for I anticipate your fierce expression when I open the door. And secondly you believe I should have such empathy that I respond to your wishes without your telling me what they are.'

I had expected that Bettina might challenge me on these examples but she agreed the substance of them. She then told me of an urge to burrow inside me and get into a 'heavenly place, a sort of Garden of Eden', asking me if I draw away from her (as she believes I do when she is needy) because of this. I said I thought not.

There are, of course, many issues that could be explored when recounting this kind of interchange. I am concerned here, for the most part, with the issue of what is reasonable and what is proper for Bettina and I to ask of each other, give to each other, and refuse to give to each other. These are real, present day matters between two people who, among other things are trying to co-operate yet anxious to preserve their own identity and integrity. The fact that the transference and countertransference issues inherent in a helping situation profoundly affect what is going on does not invalidate the actual, present day endeavour and struggle.

Even with hindsight I do not know whether Bettina's criticism of me was justified or not. The reason for relating this interchange is less to find an answer to that issue than to explore the way in which the disagreement between us can be usefully conceived. If it were simply a matter of my knowledge (through experience and theory) of a correct way, as an expert, to respond to her distress, then it would be equivalent to giving penicillin for pneumonia. But the equivalence, in this case, is better portrayed by the parent who has to find a response to a child who is frightened or bewildered. The child's distress may be of such magnitude that she is unable to act morally: she cannot extricate herself from her anguish but can, perhaps, be comforted. Insofar as she is asking for care she is asking for a response that is appropriate. On the other hand, her request may be a move in a battle for power for its own sake. The parent, using his knowledge of the child, his intuition, and his philosophy of living will act (if he acts with good intent) in the way that seems best to him. I believe the same applies to therapist and patient. But the fact that the patient, in the process of seeking help, may often feel more like a child than she does in many situations, does not necessarily take away her moral responsibility nor preclude the therapist from acting on the basis of his moral beliefs.

It is all too easy, however, to press a viewpoint beyond its valid reach. Morality, even when given a broad definition, is only applicable in a situation in which a person is responsible for their action. Even if we attribute a capacity for choice to an infant from the earliest times, his power to use this capacity is very limited. He needs (as Erikson emphasizes so strongly) to be able to trust; but he can only do so appropriately if the setting is trustworthy. If this is lacking there is little he can do about it, and, as an adult in therapy he is in no position to manufacture an appropriate trust; it can only grow. Lacking this trust he will not be able to respond with the degree of responsibility that we expect of people in ordinary life. To estimate this degree, and have expectations that are appropriate is, to my mind, as difficult a task as we are likely to face as therapists.

It is the recognition of the vulnerability and frailty of the infant, and of some adults who later come for help, that is the centre of Winnicott's work. The response that is required is, in

certain cases, like that of the mother of a small child, one of devoted care. Implicitly, Winnicott takes the responsibility of the
task on his shoulders, relying on his intuitive capacity to know
when this is appropriate. The risk of infantilization is great and
depends on how well the two people manage to share the responsibility for the endeavour and are aware of the limitations
of their own moral beliefs.

There is a significant difference, from the moral point of
view, between the situation of the therapist who is faced, from
the beginning, with someone who is disintegrated and needs to
be 'held', and that of the psychoanalyst who believes that his
treatment inevitably, if only temporarily, leads to an incapacity
to make realistic judgements. This is one of the dilemmas
which Hinchelwood addresses in a very thoughtful book on
the dangers of coercion by psychoanalysis.[2] The vulnerability
of the patient, he believes, is heightened by the phenomenon
of the transference fostered by psychoanalytic technique. He
notes that 'the patient consents to a collusion that dismantles
his coherent personality. He cannot make his decisions out of
a proper balance of mind'.[3] To the extent that this is the case in
analysis the danger of unwitting coercion are, indeed, formidable. In seeking to justify this risk, Hinchelwood argues that
psychoanalytic understanding will, in the end, combat the
danger of undue influence—an optimism that I find difficult to
share. This does not mean, of course, that those of us who do
not practise psychoanalytic technique cannot get help from
Freud's insights in a way that may assist in our struggle to do
justice to the patient's experience. I will give an example.

Ruby's recovery from a breakdown was extraordinarily slow
and she seemed, at times, to be quite stuck. I alternated between simply supporting her in the hope that growth would
occur, and encouraging, or even provoking, her to take more
risks.

One day she brought a dream.

I had just lit a small fire. It was a bit to one side of the grate. Someone
came into the room and said the fire should be in the middle of the
grate and started to move it. But I prevented this, saying "It's not got
going enough yet to move it. If you do that it will go out".

In view of all I knew about her the dream seemed to suggest
that she needed to grow at her own pace. I had to rely on my

intuition—and hers—for this interpretation, for I know there are other possibilities, but I was grateful for what seemed a nudge in the right direction. I would not say that I followed Freud's technique of dream analysis but I used his insight that dreams contain symbolic meanings.

I will now return to Bettina. I wrote the above description of my conversations with her at the time that the interchange occurred. A couple of years after the therapy had ended I showed it to her and we discussed my opinions at some length. Although the account seemed to her to be more or less factually correct as far as she could remember she disagreed with some of the ways in which I had interpreted them. There was, she felt, no chance of a harmful infantilization although she did agree that she was reliving a childhood struggle, namely, a need to preserve her identity against the pull of her own parents' dependency on her. Now, she told me, she realizes that she is a more independent person by nature than we had recognized at the time. I think that she was probably right. She now lives a life in which she is comfortable in her own position in relation to others and there is no evidence of undue dependence.

Certainly, in the room with her now there was no trace of any fear of or unease with me. Indeed, it felt rather strange to be debating the differences between us which had caused such anguish at the time yet could now be confronted with mutual calm.

On reflection, I think that my original interpretation of events contained an element of defensiveness in that I saw Bettina as more of an insatiable child than was the case; rather, it was the terror of losing integrity that led her to challenge me in ways that threatened my own perceptions. 'It was,' she now said, 'indeed a moral struggle. It was between my need to protect myself and my desire not to hurt you.' She made another observation. 'I feel you were not ordinary enough. In ordinary life you would smile at someone who comes to your house, you would probably be more accommodating about the window, if only out of courtesy. I feel that, because of a theory or technique, you felt you needed to have your way.'

I am still not sure about the validity of her comment on this point. But I have to confess that, if we could then have achieved the ordinary, friendly atmosphere of this later meeting I may well have acted with more generosity.

One way of formulating the dilemma I have addressed here is to say that it is important to give due respect to the patient's judgement as an equal human being yet to recognize and even focus on the failures of his judgement. This is no easy task. Even if the therapist is prepared to admit to mistakes of judgement when it is appropriate to do so, the focus will inevitably fall on the patient's limitations. Balance could only be obtained if, following Ferenczi, we practised mutual analysis; but, except perhaps in exceptional circumstances, this seems to be carrying an ideal beyond the realms of common sense. When it comes to writing about therapy the scales appear to be even more tipped in the therapist's favour. The therapist does not write about himself; he writes about those who come to him. One way in which he could disclose his imperfect judgements would be to publish an account of his own personal therapy, but it may not happen to be very interesting and carries the danger of indulgence in narcissism. And, in my case, it would also be thirty years too late. It is with a recognition of this limitation that I now give an account of a patient's dream in order to illustrate her difficulty in maintaining her own judgement in the face of authority.

A woman told me that over the past few days she had been very disturbed and was wondering whether she was 'mad or bad'. This state of mind had been precipitated by an argument with a friend; the rights and wrongs of the matter seemed to hinge on such intangibles as the tone of voice in which comments had been made. This kind of conflict, so familiar to those who are close to each other, precipitated the following dream.

I was back in childhood. We were moving to a new house and I was very excited. There was a room each for my sister and myself and we were all pleased with what we'd got. My sister had a smaller room but it was pretty and interesting, and she liked it. Then we seemed to be going to the house again, but this time the small room was quite different—shabby, dirty, and uninteresting. Nobody could like such a room. I knew with a sinking heart that it would be allotted to me and that I would accept it.

Does the dream depict an acceptance of the necessity of coming to terms with reality or a resigned, defeated recognition of an unfair situation in which one's voice will inevitably be ignored? How can the child judge? The dream seemed to confirm that she had grown up with a disabling incapacity to assess the validity of her stance in life and a warning to me that I must be careful not to influence her unduly.

Someone who suffers some degree of defeat in childhood and later comes for therapy will inevitably have a sense of shame, and perhaps guilt, on account of their failure. She has not fulfilled her potential and has not been true to herself. She has, moreover, not been true to others. In order to survive and adapt to the world she has deceived those around her, if not herself, as to her true nature. She may, for example, be unduly co-operative and self-effacing; or she may pretend to a competence and independence which is more of an act than the genuine article. To either maintain or abandon a false position may require courage, albeit of a different kind in each case. It clearly takes unusual nerve to be a spy, always under threat of exposure; yet it also requires courage to confess and take the consequences. The same dilemma applies to the homosexual who may or may not decide to 'come out'.

There are many factors which contribute towards the moment when someone may drop a defence: the intellectual insight she may gain from an appropriate interpretation; an increase of trust in the therapist; a gathering strength over a period of therapy; or an illuminating or encouraging happening in her ordinary life. She is not, however, a passive automaton, entirely subject to the forces pressing upon her, and therefore choice and courage will play a part in the outcome. In other words, the decision will, in part, be a moral one and depend on her moral stance in the world: what she believes to be the good life and the degree to which she will strive to attain it. Finally—and perhaps most difficult of all—she needs to face and resist the temptation to use her weakness in order to manipulate others.

How should the therapist respond to these matters? How can he estimate the degree to which self-expression should flourish? If this includes wanton destructiveness, are we to sit back and encourage this? How should he conceive the 'true self'? An id-like, Darwinian, ruthless greed that must be tamed and suppressed, or a reasonable drive to exist, to explore, to experience, capable of both ruthlessness or concern, but, at the beginning, lost, unlearned, needing direction from without? Such different emphases will affect his therapeutic approach, and will have a bearing on how he judges the relative rights of parent and child, therapist and patient.

When two people, let us say, husband and wife, become familiar with psychoanalytic ideas their rows take on a new and more formidable dimension. Both are tempted to interpret the other's point of view in order to undermine it. If, however, the marriage was constructed in such a way that only one of them was given the authority to interpret and to conceal his thoughts, feelings, and actions from the other, the consequences are too awful to contemplate. Yet the technique which is held as a model, not only for psychoanalysts, but for many of those who work in the fields of psychotherapy or counselling, depicts a situation that is uncomfortably close to the hypothetical marriage I describe. And even those who do not subscribe to a technique of this kind will find it difficult, by virtue of accepting the role of a helper rather than simply a friend, to avoid using their position to impose a moral judgement in their favour.

References

1. Margolit, A. (1996). *The decent society*, (trans. N. Goldblum). Harvard University Press, Cambridge, MA.
2. Hinchelwood, R. D. (1997). *Therapy or coercion? Does psychoanalysis differ from brainwashing?* Karnac, London.
3. Ibid. p. 100.

10

Fragmentation, psychotherapy, and society

Everything that happens is as normal and expected as the spring rose or the summer fruit; this is true of sickness, death, slander, intrigue, and all the other things that delight or trouble foolish men.
Marcus Aurelius

The loss of vitality and the distortion of truth which occurs when morality is excluded from a dialogue about human experience has been noted by so many thinkers in the past that any selection is bound to be arbitrary. In the field of literature Wordsworth and Coleridge are pre-eminent. In an essay on Wordsworth, Matthew Arnold writes of the 'noble and profound' application of ideas to life and the application of those ideas under the conditions fixed for us by the laws of poetic beauty or poetic truth:

If it is said that to call these ideas moral ideas is to introduce a strong and injurious limitation, I answer that it is to do nothing of the kind because moral ideas are really so main a part of human life. The question, how to live, is itself a moral idea; and it is the question which most interests every man, and with which, in some way or other, he is perpetually occupied. A large sense is of course to be given to the term moral. Whatever bears upon the question, "how to live", comes under it.[1]

If we are to use the term 'moral' in the meaning it had for Arnold it becomes clear that the situation of literary criticism today is under an even greater threat than in his time of failing to appreciate the centrality of the question 'How should we live?' As Stephen Logan puts it:

For the first time in literary history the bulk of serious criticism is devoid of moral content. Read almost any essay by a major British critic from, say, Dryden to Arnold and you'll find unmistakable evidence of a belief that most people who read at all seriously do so from moral motives. This belief, if not explicitly stated, will be implicit in the critic's entire manner of address. Readers, it was assumed wanted help in finding out how to live. They read poems, romances and plays, as well as the more obviously informative kinds of literature, in search of wisdom. They turned to critics in the hope of refining their moral reactions to what they had read. In our own time, however, critics venture upon moral questions reluctantly and with embarrassment—as if declaring their moral concerns proved them "unsophisticated", and intellectual sophistication were the highest good.

By eliminating the moral dimension of their work, academic critics ensure that they are read not in the hope of enlightenment—as our predecessors would have read Johnson or Hazlitt—but at best with respect for a relatively barren cleverness.[2]

In this book I have tried to convey my conviction that there is a lack of serious discussion of morality in the field of psychotherapy comparable to that in literature noted by Logan, with the consequence that the illumination which people search for is often dimmed by unnecessary and inappropriate technical measures.

The large questions about life are beyond our comprehension; we cannot get a direct grasp on them. But we can, often with amazing accuracy and with marvellous results, form conceptions of less complex problems. In this respect we are like computers—or perhaps it would be better to say that we are somewhere between a computer and a God. Tempted by our incredible technical abilities we tackle the world piecemeal. Sometimes, these pieces can be put together and give us new illuminations. But we pay a price, and the price is fragmentation.

In his book *Wholeness and the implicate order*,[3] David Bohm states that,

. . . fragmentation is now very widespread, not only in society but also in each individual: and this is leading to a general confusion of the mind, which creates an endless series of problems and interferes with our clarity of perception so seriously as to prevent us from being able to solve most of them.

Thus, art, science, technology, and human work in general are divided up into specialities, each considered to be separate in essence from the others. Becoming dissatisfied with this state of affairs men have set up further interdisciplinary subjects which were intended to unite these specialities, but these new subjects have ultimately served mainly to add further separate fragments'.[3]

Bohm draws on Aristotle's notion of 'formal cause', translating it into more modern language as 'an ordered and structured inner movement that is essential to what things are'. This implies a 'final cause', which may be brought about by conscious design but more usually:

Men often aim towards certain ends in their thoughts but what actually emerges from their actions is generally something different from what was in their design, something that was, however, implicit in what they were doing, though not consciously perceived by those who took part.[4]

In Bohm's view, however, we have now, particularly in the West, 'extended the process of division beyond the limits within which it works properly'. Although most of his argument is derived from theoretical physics he makes quite clear his conviction that our contemporary ways of thinking about living in general are grossly disturbed by our assumption that the world is made up of separate entities. This fixed belief is so powerful, he notes, that even those working in the field of quantum mechanics fail to recognize the implications of their discoveries. We cannot, however, now return to the thinking of the remote past, nor can we, in a makeshift way, piece together what we have already separated:

What is called for is not an *integration* of thought, or a kind of imposed unity, for any such imposed point of view would itself be merely another fragment. Rather, all our different ways of thinking are to be considered as different ways of looking at the one reality, each with some domain in which it is clear and adequate.[5]

Psychotherapists vary greatly in their reliance either on an intuitive, open-ended approach or on the formation of a plan based on logical thinking. Freudian analysts veer towards the former (although they do not usually put it this way); cognitive therapists, and most practitioners who use short-term methods, prefer the latter. As in so many matters, Freud's position is ambiguous. Working in the nineteenth-century scientific tradition he produced theories based on the cataloguing of discrete entities, instincts, defences, complexes, stages of development, etc. His explanations incorporated not only the disintegration that occurs in a disturbed person but what he considered to be the normal and natural state of human beings. And many of his followers have formulated theories which rival his atomization of ordinary experience. Yet, it was Freud who enabled us to recognize the capacity of the unconscious to abolish our conscious tendency to compartmentalize life and who advocated a method by means of which ('free-floating attention') we can most easily allow this unconscious function to emerge. The concept of 'countertransference', by means of which we understand the state of the other person by becoming aware of our own is close to what we might call 'intuition'. For these reasons, psychoanalysis has turned out to be a confusing mixture of wholeness and fragmentation, technique and empathy. Insofar as it involves the gradual unfolding and understanding of a relationship occurring in an atmosphere of freedom and tolerance and a respect for the unknown it is an endeavour conducive to the healing of dissociation. And many, if not most, psychoanalysts have been inspired by Freud's teachings to adopt a stance of receptivity akin to Keat's description of 'negative capability'. Yet there remains a curious split.

Wilfrid Bion is one of the most celebrated psychoanalysts of recent years and his advice that the analyst should approach his patient in a state of mind that is 'without memory or desire'[6] has become famous; he speaks strongly in favour of openness and willingness to be surprised, allowing the feelings of the patient free access to himself. Bion's phrase, 'without memory and desire', is a poetic one; I doubt if we should, or can, take it literally. But as I suggested earlier, it is clear that many analysts do practise in this way, laying themselves open to the pain of the patient, often at great emotional cost to themselves;

the moving accounts of Harold Searles[7] are a striking example of this. Yet, as Frosch notes, in reference to Bion's ideas:

This is not necessarily the way in which the psychoanalytic movement presents itself to the world. Not all psychoanalytic learning is aimed at freeing the analyst from preconceptions; on the contrary, psychoanalysis makes many truth claims concerned, for example, with the mechanisms of the mind, the cause of human development, the causes of psychological distress and the vicissitudes of sexuality.[8]

We are certainly dealing here with a failure on the part of psychoanalysts to describe coherently what they do. To what extent preconceptions interfere with their capacity to receive openly (to free themselves from the role of expert) is hard to know; sometimes, I think, they do what they intuitively feel is right and be damned of the consequences. Recently, a colleague described her response to a patient who was faced with an appalling and dreadful occurrence in the actual world. She cancelled her day's work and went to him. 'I broke all the rules,' she said, 'I couldn't do anything else. But I felt bad about it afterwards. I wondered if I could go on with the analysis after that, but he insisted.' I feel that what she had done was brave, humane, and therapeutic but I was momentarily surprised that she could think her action would do anything other than enhance the therapy.

The concept of countertransference has an ambiguous relation to that of negative capability. The therapist, in letting herself be open to the patient, can become conscious of feelings of which she herself was not hitherto aware. In recognizing this phenomenon she can then understand something that is deeply repressed by the patient and use this understanding to give him insight. Although the process can be explained in ordinary language the word 'countertransference' is a useful and quick way of calling one's attention to something that might well have been missed. There is a danger, however, that in separating transference and countertransference as attributes of patient and analyst, respectively, one may be making an undue distinction between the partners, for each will intuitively respond to the other in ways that are sometimes distorted by unconscious fantasy yet sometimes uncannily accurate. Moreover, a focus on these mechanisms may detract from the kind of receptive attitude that is most desirable.

A cognitive account of psychotherapy is like an opera without the music. Yet those of us who deplore this aridity have ourselves little music to offer and lack the tongues of angels to convey the pathos and the passion. In striving to describe the transcendent in therapy I find myself floundering, like many others, in words and phrases ('wholeness', 'meaningful', 'human', 'sharing', 'being', etc.), which lack clear definition and have often, through too easy usage, become debased coinage. Recently, when talking to a colleague, I used the phrase 'whole person'. He exploded at me. 'It doesn't *mean* anything to say whole person. A person is a person is a person. You can't have *half* a person unless he's dead. The phrase reminds me of my grandfather's love of treacle.' It was a striking comparison. The treacle that can flow from the parson's 'holy' voice can very easily flow, with a different cadence, from the psychotherapist and counsellor.

Psychotherapy has sometimes been considered a form of teaching. This sounds a presumptuous juxtaposition if education is regarded as the imparting of information, for the therapist does not necessarily know more than her patient. But teaching is not and has not always been thought of in this way. Some of the seminal thinkers in the field of education—Dewey and Froebel, for example—saw the function of the teacher as the provider of an environment and a response which enabled the child to make the best use of his potential, to develop his own individuality, and to satisfy his natural curiosity in the world. Today, Jerome Brunner, deriving his ideas from the close observation of infants, is perhaps foremost in calling attention to children's passionate curiosity and, consequently, the importance in education of bringing out what is potentially there rather than adding something.[9] Looked at in this light the two professions—if such they be—have much in common. And the teacher can, like the therapist, also fall foul of language. The term 'permissive education' calls to mind, for many people, all sorts of treacle. What do we mean by 'educating the child for living?', or 'educating the child as a whole'? On the other hand, we all know what is meant by the three Rs. Despite the aforementioned difficulty of the word 'whole', it is hard to avoid using it when considering an education which eschews narrow didacticism in favour of addressing the child's life potentialities, whose aim is general and unspecialized, and does not impose a world view external to the child's experience or present isolated bits and pieces of 'knowledge'.

This approach to education has fallen into disrepute of late, even though some of its features have, without due acknowledgement, been absorbed into contemporary practice. Most of the debate concerning its merits or demerits centres on the accusation that such an approach fails to equip the child for the 'real' world and does not confront him with the necessity to restrain his appetites and accept discipline. Whatever the justification or not for such allegations (and this will depend to a large extent on the quality of the teacher) it obscures the main message of Froebel and those who share a similar philosophical view, namely, that education at its best is concerned with the potential of the child and that this involves his moral development. What happens in our schools today is fragmentation. There are loud and even vociferous calls for moral education but this is usually seen as a matter that is separate from ordinary learning; rather, the imposition of a code of practice, sometimes based on religious dogma, which is issued by a higher authority. In fact, there can be no such thing as didactic moral education, for education in the richest sense of the word always implies the question 'How should we live?' If the child is viewed in his complexity what is seen will include his moral vision. If this vision is short-circuited by dogmatic teaching the consequence will be moral incoherence.

Contemporary psychotherapy is not, I think, as narrow as this. Patients are not—as yet—legally subjected to cognitive tests deemed to show evidence of improvement; the aim is not to obtain the equivalent of an A-level pass. But we are moving in that direction. The papers on psychotherapy to be found in the *British Journal of Psychiatry*, for example, primarily consist of attempts to find psychological entities by means of which a course of psychotherapy can be measured. If Method A produces people who do better on a particular item (or collection of items) than Method B, then the former is pronounced superior: there is no mention of morality and no examination of the examiners about their own moral vision. We have not always looked at 'measure' in this atomistic, crude, and rigid way. For the Greeks, measure referred to the capacity to give matters their due proportion in the context of total experience; it was considered to be essential for the good life.

Earlier in this book I suggested that contemporary psychotherapy had lost its direction on account of its departure from
the ordinary, and I discussed various ways in which this had
occurred. The conception of psychotherapy as a specialized
undertaking and the emphasis on its separateness from daily
living is one aspect of the fragmentation of society. In a society
that is whole there will be an intrinsic equilibrium; sections of
the society will not be neglected or subjugated by other sections. I am not concerned here with the gross and manifest
evils that occur in societies as a consequence of the abuse of
power. I wish, rather, to restrict the discussion to the 'professionals'. The layman is ambivalent towards the professional:
he turns to her in need, often has exaggerated confidence in
her capacities, yet is very ready to criticize failure. It is when
the professional is seen as essentially dissimilar to the man-in-
the-street that the ambivalence is most apparent. The dentist,
for example, is usually conceived as different from others only
in the acquisition of a certain skill. The psychotherapist is
another matter. Although, like the dentist, she is presumed to
have acquired a particular skill, she takes on a task which implicitly makes an enormous claim: that of healing the being of
another. This sets her apart: she must be either a sage or a
charlatan. If it were more readily recognized that what she
does is essentially of the same nature as the help we give each
other at our best in ordinary living the ambivalence would, I
think, be less. What are usually singled out for note, both by
herself and society are, however, the ways in which she might
be different rather than the ways she needs to draw on her ordinary qualities.

It is understandable that society would wish to be protected from incompetent and immoral practitioners in any
field, and therefore insist that psychotherapy should emulate
professions, such as medicine, and organize itself into a group
whose members are seen to possess an acceptable degree of
skill and moral responsibility. The consequent formation of a
Registration of Psychotherapists has, however, failed to bring
the benefits that were hoped for. Criteria of excellence have
been applied that are abysmally inappropriate to psychotherapy.

When two people meet in a situation of goodwill and
mutual respect they will watch each other in order to facilitate

communication; they will focus their senses in the hope of understanding why the other person speaks and acts in a certain way: what they mean and what they are trying to say but cannot adequately formulate. This will be done with benevolent intent. This kind of watchfulness is of particular importance in psychotherapy. We may, however, watch each other for less charitable reasons. We may watch for the purpose of achieving control or in order to protect ourselves. This much is clear. What is confusing, however, is a situation in which watching is presented as altruistic, yet, consciously or unconsciously, is motivated by fear or a narcissistic urge to control. It follows that any benevolent undertaking, such as child-rearing, education, or psychotherapy, which involves an inequality of power, should be regarded with circumspection. Although we can often make an intuitive assessment of whether we are in the presence of benevolence or not the seductive power of apparent goodwill, intellectual argument or sheer force of dogmatic conviction may outweigh our perceptive abilities.

In contemporary society most people are no longer in fear of the omniscience of God or find themselves regarded of sufficient importance that their homes are bugged. Yet there is a rapidly accelerating centralized knowledge of what we are up to, partly due to the improved technical methods of surveillance, and partly due to a widespread belief that the more we know about the activities of people the better society can be organized for good and protected from bad. And it can hardly be doubted that such knowledge can be of use as, for example, the notification of typhoid carriers. We need to question, however, whether there is a threshold beyond which surveillance is harmful, in what sort of cases it may be inappropriate, and the degree to which it is benign.

It would be of benefit if psychotherapists who are so morally corrupt that they constitute a grave threat to those who seek their help were made known to the public; the danger is comparable to that of a typhoid carrier who works in a restaurant. Public health authorities usefully extend their concerns and powers far beyond the matter of typhoid. There are increasing checks and regulations to try to ensure that those who eat out will not be poisoned—and we have reason to be grateful for such rational measures, even though we may become concerned if the measures appear to reach obsessional degrees or are ill conceived, or unprincipled. But what of psychotherapy? Should we similarly give our approval to a corresponding set of regulations?

The matter of typhoid is a relatively clear one. The bacillus can be identified in the body and a certain dose of antibiotic will destroy it in large, if not always sufficient numbers; the treatment is accepted by the medical profession, and is given a blessing by most of the population. Psychotherapy is, in this respect, a different matter. There is no generally agreed definition of the troubles which people bring to their therapists and no general agreement as to how these troubles can be relieved. Thus, psychotherapists inhabit an uncertain world. In Britain, those who wish to practise choose a technique and attend a training scheme that specializes in this particular technique. If they succeed in convincing their teachers that they have become competent in the technique then they can officially practise psychotherapy. The teachers themselves—or, rather, the group of teachers who collectively teach the technique— have to convince a central power that they are competent to teach and that the technique they espouse is a satisfactory method of healing. Those approaches which can lay claim to conform to the widespread respect for 'scientific method' are more likely to be considered valuable. One begins to wonder whether the whole operation amounts to much more than an exercise in public relations, rather as a divided government may seek to portray itself as a unified organization.

In the United States, psychotherapy is organized in quite a different way to that of Britain but the underlying trend is the same. Although much more of the funding of medical and mental health care comes from insurance companies these are regulated by the state. In an article entitled 'Mental healing under managed care',[10] Nathaniel Pallone deplores the degree to which chemical remedies for emotional distress are replacing the 'talking cure' because of legal restraints based on 'cost-effectiveness' as well as the power of advertisement. The threat to the talking cure (the kind of therapy or counselling about which I write) comes also from the claims for respectability by cognitive psychology. Thomas Szasz,[11] in noting this trend, quotes the President of the National Association for Consumer Protection on Mental Health Practices:

Consumers will now have to be told that psychotherapists who want to talk about the patients' childhood are offering them what is . . . possibly a harmful procedure. Just as importantly the modern, scientifically based treatment, such as cognitive, behavioural treatments must now, according to the law, be explicitly offered to all psychotherapy patients suffering from depression and anxiety.

The tendency for insurance companies to insist that cognitive–behavioural methods are the only acceptable psychological interventions has, unhappily, now passed over to Britain,[12] the psychotherapist who works independently is currently little affected by this. The danger of being coerced into conformity of some kind stems from the health service and the process of registration. If we think that, with time, creative work within the registration process will be virtually impossible we will advise prospective students to have nothing to do with it and seek to learn how to help people outside the system. If, however, we are less pessimistic, we will search for means of limiting the intrusiveness of standardized methods of teaching and monitoring practice. I find it difficult to foresee how the latter can be achieved without a paradigm shift. If psychotherapy can be seen to be a personal matter then it becomes clear that we are dealing with an intimate relationship and that the restrictions on the privacy of such a relationship have to be viewed with the utmost caution. There is a quality to some relationships—those, for example, between friends, lovers, and family members—which, in any society that deserves to be called civilized, is respected as primarily a private matter. We would, I imagine, think it wrong to legislate the positions in which people make love or the words and gestures with which parents communicate with their children, or whether friends should meet in each other's houses or in a pub. The relationship which develops in good psychotherapy has, I believe, a comparable quality of intimacy and uniqueness, and is not amenable to standardization. It is a long time since Heraclitus made the point: 'If one does not expect the unexpected, one will not find it out, untrackable as it is pathless'.

The nature of psychotherapy has always reflected the beliefs of the society of its time, and the way mainstream psychotherapy is now is an expression of the way society is now. The emphasis on performance, efficiency, and standardization is an outcome of the industrial age, inevitably squeezing out personal autonomy.

The loss of autonomy has been accompanied by a loss of the sense of responsibility to others: an atrophy of civic virtue. In place of what might have once been considered as an aspect of the natural order of civilized living—the mutual support given, however imperfectly, by family and friends—we increasingly turn to paid professionals for succour. Psychotherapists need to be aware that in fulfilling this function they may, implicitly and unwittingly, denigrate and erode the capacities of ordinary people to help those in emotional turmoil.

The invasiveness of medical and therapeutic techniques has been outlined by many writers, including Rieff,[13] Foucault,[14] Donzelot,[15] Illich,[16] Lasch,[17] Ingleby,[18] and Smail[19]. According to Lasch, from the late nineteenth-century onwards:

> Doctors, psychiatrists, social workers, child guidance experts and other experts derided maternal instinct, home remedies and rule-of-thumb methods, claiming to substitute for the traditional love of women new techniques based on science "understood only by those with professional training".

This critique has not, for the most part, been seen as an attack on ordinariness, wholeness, or goodness, but much of it can be conceived in these terms.

The respect for ordinariness diminishes with every new technique. Medical expertise has much evidence to justify its methods (although less than is commonly supposed), and the cultural impact of this fact puts increasing pressure on the therapist to think and practise under the guidance of a centralized organization, rather than rely on the quality of their relationship with those who seek help.

References

1. Arnold, Mathew (1911). *Essays in Criticism*, p. 142. MacMillan, London.
2. Logan, S. (Personal communication.)
3. Bohm, D. (1980). *Wholeness and the implicit order*. Routledge, London.
4. Ibid., p. 13.

5. Ibid., pp. 7, 8.
6. Bion, W. (1970). *Attention and interpretation*. Tavistock, London.
7. Searles, H. (1965). *Papers on schizophrenia and related subjects*. Hogarth/Institute of Psychoanalysis, London.
8. Frosch, S. (1997). *For and against psychoanalysis*, p. 15. Routledge, London.
9. Bruner, J. (1990). *Acts of meaning*, Harvard University Press, Cambridge, MA.
10. Pallone, N. J. (1997). Mental healing under managed care. *Society*, **35**, 8–17.
11. Szasz, T. (1999). Discretion as power: In the situation called psychotherapy. *British Journal of Psychotherapy*, **15**, 216–29.
12. Lomas, P. (1999). Response to Szasz. *British Journal of Psychotherapy*, **15**, 370–1.
13. Reiff, P. (1987). *The triumph of the therapeutic*. University of Chicago.
14. Foucault, M. (1979) *The history of sexuality*. Vol. i: An Introduction (trans. R. Harley). Allen Lane, London.
15. Donzelot, J. (1980). *The policing of families*, (trans. R. Harley). Hutchinson, London.
16. Illich, I. (1976). *Limits to medicine*. Marion Boyers, London.
17. Ingleby, D. (1983). Mental health and social order. In *Social control and the state*, (eds. S. Cohen and A. Scull). Martin Robertson, London.
18. Lasch, L. (1980). *New York Review of Books*, 12 June, p. 27.
19. Smail, D. (1996). *How to survive without psychotherapy*. Constable, London.

Index